If I Only Had a Brain Injury

If I Only Had a Brain Injury

A TBI Survivor and Life Coach's Guide to
Chronic Fatigue, Concussion, Lyme Disease,
Migraine or Other "Medical Mystery"

Laura Bruno, M.A.

To order additional copies of this book, contact:
Xlibris Corporation
1-888-795-4274
www.Xlibris.com
Orders@Xlibris.com
46578

Contents

About the Cover Photo 11
Acknowledgements 13

"Somewhere Over the Rainbow" 15

"We're Not in Kansas Anymore" 19

Glinda 26
1. Contact organizations and support groups 27
2. Have a neuropsychological evaluation 30
3. Consult a behavioral optometrist 32
4. Try CranioSacral therapy 34
5. Get evaluated for Lyme Disease 36
6. Choose your lawyer carefully 41

Ruby Slippers and the Wicked Witch of the West 44
7. Forgive yourself for taking so long to recover 46
8. Recognize parts that needed to change 48
9. Draw upon what you already know 49
10. Follow your intuition 51

"Follow the Yellow Brick Road" 53
11. Buy top quality electronics 54
12. Find ways to minimize stimulation 56
13. Breathe slowly and fully 58
14. Do the cross-crawl 60
15. Practice yoga 62
16. Search for patterns 65

"If I Only Had a Brain" 66
17. Cultivate relationships with animals 67
18. Initiate new friendships 69
19. Practice Mindfulness 72
20. Listen to classical music 73
21. Listen to books and lectures on tape 74

Crabby Apple Trees 75
22. Check any medications for side effects 76
23. Buy "Organic." 77
24. "Let your food be your medicine." 79
25. Learn to utilize natural remedies 85
26. Consider a Candida connection 89
27. Indulge your senses—but not all at once 91

"If I Only Had a Heart" 92
28. Find a balance in intimate relationships 93
29. Laugh more 96
30. Celebrate 98
31. Learn to live from your heart & let go 99

"Courage" 101
32. Write a letter to your pain 102
33. Relinquish your attachment to recovery 103
34. Express your vulnerability 104
35. Try something new 105
36. Don't be afraid to pursue your dreams 107

Poppies and Sudden Snow Showers 108
37. Don't distract as you approach goals 109
38. Get plenty of sleep 110
39. Record your dreams 111
40. Pray—with gratitude 113

"Surrender Dorothy" 115
41. Don't take it personally 116
42. Not everyone wants you to recover 117
43. Practice patience 118
44. Setbacks often precede big steps forward 120

Melting the Wicked Witch 123
45. Hold a funeral service for your "old self." 124
46. Forgive whoever caused your injury 126
47. Choose recovery AND financial security 127
48. Quit looking for shortcuts 132

The Wonderful Wizard of Oz 134
49. Create a sacred space for yourself 135
50. Listen to Pink Floyd's Dark Side of the Moon 137

51. Look for the bigger picture 138
52. Be yourself 139

Epilogue 141

Appendix 1: "Glinda's Secrets"
    (A Special Section for Treatment Providers) 143

Appendix 2: "Aunty Em!"
    (A Special Section for Caregivers) 153

Appendix 3: "We Welcome You to Munchkin Land"
    (Survivors Share their Stories) 173

To Stephen, with love.

About the Cover Photo

My husband, Stephen, took this photograph of a boulder on November 13, 2007 in Sedona, Arizona. When he loaded it into the computer, we noticed that the shadows had formed a descending "hand." At first, it reminded me of Michelangelo's famous "Hand of God" reaching to touch Adam's finger on The Sistine Chapel ceiling, but when I looked at the photo again, the hand seemed to be gently reaching *into a brain*!

   I had pondered various cover images for a long time, and this photo captures what so many survivors experience as a deeper sense of meaning and purpose behind their trauma. May each of you discover this touch of the Divine . . .

Acknowledgements

I offer heartfelt thanks to all the contributors to this book: Robin Bernhard, Robin Cohn, Professor Stephen Hawking, Sandra K. Heggen, Stephanie Jellison, Sarah Kramer, Terri Nelson, Dr. William Padula, Rev. Daniel Prechtel, Sandy Rakowitz, the late Dana Reeve, Karen Ruppert, and Kay Strom.

Special thanks to Sally Kempton, Lyn Miller-Lachmann, Sarah Moore and Patricia Spork for reading and offering your suggestions on key portions of this project.

I'd also like to thank all the people who made possible my "miraculous" recovery, especially Dr. George N. Dever, Dr. Jeffery Getzell, Attorney Mike Gillick, Wendy Madgwick, and Dr. Joseph Sataloff. My recovery involved so many people that I cannot possibly name you all. To anyone who drove me to appointments, shared a laugh, prayed for me, and/or believed that I could heal, many thanks and blessings!

Most of all, I thank my husband, Stephen Bruno, for never treating me like a disabled person, always believing in my dreams and for challenging me to live them.

"Somewhere Over the Rainbow"

I *understand* the physical and emotional toll exacted by sudden dependence on other people, misdiagnoses, insurance restrictions, legal battles, and a society that does not recognize your symptoms.

I know how it feels to go from "high achiever" to "below average" and have doctors tell you to feel grateful. I realize how body and brain can become so fatigued that you cannot possibly get out of bed—even though you just slept sixteen hours.

I understand, because on May 19, 1998 a car accident destroyed the life I knew. Traumatic brain injury (TBI) replaced my sales career and graduate school fellowship. Instead of tangible bonuses or grades, I spent the next six years chasing elusive *Recovery*.

According to one clinician who treats TBI, Fibromyalgia, Multiple Chemical Sensitivities, and Chronic Fatigue Syndrome, "Most people reach a comfortable state of disability and then quit."

He admired me for persevering, even when doctors told me I would never read longer than twenty minutes per day. He praised my determination to tolerate florescent lights again. He told me I must possess amazing willpower to continue searching for treatments.

This clinician might have known how people typically respond to trauma, but he certainly did not understand my motivation to recover. Simply put, I hated being injured. *I wanted my life back.*

Actually, I wanted more than that. I had missed my mid-to-late-twenties; I wanted a new life that was so good, it helped make up for what I'd lost. As long as I could *imagine* a better life, I would not resign myself to quitting. I felt compelled to reach for something more.

If I Only Had a Brain Injury is for the other *Wizard of Oz* fans of this world: for the dreamers. For those who dare ask, "Why oh why . . . can't I?" and refuse to let ill health provide a final answer. I wrote this book for anyone who has ever wished to go "somewhere over the rainbow."

*   *   *

Frank Baum presents one of the strangest (and most famous) examples of TBI in his classic, *The Wonderful Wizard of Oz*. Hours after Dorothy wishes to go "somewhere over the rainbow," she hits her head on a window frame ripped loose by the twister.

The impact knocks her out. In the space between knock out and reawakening, Dorothy finds herself "somewhere over the rainbow." Her epic journey begins as she tries to find her way back home.

Few people recognize the centrality of brain injury in *The Wizard of Oz*, but this beloved film informed my recovery. I remember watching it the first time post-injury: "If Dorothy can find her way from Oz to Kansas, then surely I can find my way from total disability to some variety of 'real world' life."

To my blunted intellect, Dorothy's fairy tale victory seemed at least as relevant as any medical prognosis. Like Ruby Slippers magically appearing on my feet, the film lit up my mind—prompting me to find and follow a golden path to healing. As a child believes in Santa Claus, the tooth fairy, or *The Wizard of Oz*, I believed I could get well.

Dorothy begins the film by longing for something more than mere survival: "If happy little bluebirds fly, then why, oh, why, oh why can't I?" Lonely and bored, she would probably have remained a mere daydreamer were it not for the timely arrival of Miss Gulch. The angry neighbor confiscates the girl's beloved Toto.

When the dog returns home, Dorothy recognizes the impossibility of inaction. For if Miss Gulch finds Toto again, she will have him killed, and Dorothy will lose him forever.

Initially, Dorothy runs away. This action protects Toto, but Dorothy finds herself unwilling to leave her old life entirely behind. She turns back towards Auntie Em, even though nothing at home has changed.

As soon as Dorothy *Gale* abandons her resolve to leave, the winds begin. She arrives at the farm, too late to join the others in a tornado shelter.

Chance, Fate or Divine Intervention isolates the dreamer, leaving her vulnerable to a highly individual "accident."

When the twister rips a window frame from the wall and knocks her out, Dorothy receives an answer to her prayer for change. As so often happens in life—particularly to people who sustain TBI—the answer is bigger and more demanding than she thought she wanted.

But Dorothy recognizes the answer almost immediately in Munchkin Land, as she ponders, "We must be over the rainbow."

Recovery in Dorothy's case—i.e. awakening from her concussion—means returning to herself with a new perspective on the magic and compassion of everyday life. Recovery for me meant something similar.

*   *   *

As a Life Coach, Medical Intuitive and former assistant to a holistic vision and brain injury clinician in Seattle, I have aided hundreds of people dealing with life's worst nightmares. Combined with my own recovery experience, this background certainly qualified me to write *If I Only Had a Brain Injury*.

Yet in October 2004, trauma struck close to home again. My husband contracted Lyme Disease from a field mouse tick bite.

Far away from the Northeastern United States' epidemic area, we initially rationalized his symptoms as a complex blend of unrelated annoyances. However, the problems increased in severity, closely mimicking my earlier visual disturbances, headaches, fatigue and memory problems.

Numerous specialists repeated the refrain I had heard so often during my own recovery: "We just don't know what to tell you. It could be migraines, or maybe stress. Maybe you have arthritis. Maybe none of these problems is actually related. It could all be one huge coincidence. Are you depressed? You know, sometimes emotional problems cause physical symptoms."

No one offered a solution, and no one seemed to care that my husband's once active, joyful life consisted of darkened rooms, restricted activity, chronic pain and a feeling that somewhere along the way, he had "lost himself."

Recognizing my husband's struggle, and knowing all too well how it feels on the receiving end of uncertain prognoses and raised eyebrows, I accepted the mission to help him recover.

So many of the methods I had used to heal myself from TBI proved effective in treating his illness that I decided to expand my manuscript. What I had initially envisioned as purely a TBI recovery book grew into a healing guide for any injury or illness that affects one's sense of "self."

People who suffer neurological shifts will find most resonance with my story and hints, but these recommendations can be easily adapted for other types of chronic pain or illness.

The Appendices include first person essays and interviews of survivors, caregivers and treatment providers intimately familiar with a variety of illnesses and injuries. If you do not identify with my particular struggles and triumphs, then I hope you will find the words and experiences of my contributors both healing and inspirational.

The suggestions in this book are ones that helped me and helped other people with TBI, brain cancer, Fibromyalgia, Lyme Disease, vertigo, *Candida* overgrowth, and Chronic Fatigue Syndrome. They also helped clients, students and friends who found their lives suddenly turned upside down by trauma. In retrospect, these life challenges (worst nightmares) often evolved into dreams come true.

Not to say this metamorphosis was easy or exactly the way any of us would have planned! A fellow pilgrim on the road to recovery, I designed *If I Only Had a Brain Injury* to support your quest for wellness and to help you learn from and appreciate the journey.

I am required by law to tell you that I am not a doctor, and I can't promise you will make a full recovery. Nor should sharing from my own experiences and observations ever be taken as medical advice. I am a Life Coach, Medical Intuitive, Reiki Master Teacher and Writer—not a neurologist, psychologist or infectious diseases specialist!

What I *do* offer here are ideas, stories and questions that help you to receive the greatest blessings from your experience—and to embrace the greatest possible healing.

I aim to inspire you and to guide you to resources that will empower you to take control over your own health and wellbeing.

You can approach this book in a variety of ways:

1) If you prefer a narrative, the next chapter, "We're Not in Kansas Anymore," details my first few months of TBI. It gives you the original context and a sense of how far I needed to recover in order to write this book.
2) If you want to skip directly to the healing hints, turn to the chapter called "Glinda."
3) If you read straight through, you will notice that the book's structure allows you to follow your own "Yellow Brick Road" to recovery. I tell a story within a story and invite you to join the journey.
4) You can choose to read a hint a day, or one a week.
5) You can also play "Reading Roulette" and open to a "random" page, trusting synchronicity to provide you with exactly what you need.

With persistence, imagination and a warm heart, you, too, can find your way back home.

"We're Not in Kansas Anymore"

Six months before my brain injury, a nightmare stalked me:

> *I stood schmoozing at a cocktail party. Wild dog devoured my left butt cheek. I screamed, but the person babbled on. I looked around at people drinking champagne and flirting. No one noticed anything unusual. I began to laugh in sharp, shrill hyperventilation. The party carried on. I detached my mind from the pain in my body and quietly mused, "A Doberman just ate my butt." Then I moved on to the next topic of conversation, as though I became one of the other guests.*

With each recurrence, the dream intensified. Two days before my car accident, I awoke in terror, followed by giddiness. I failed to settle into the conclusion's nonchalance. Inner foreboding refrained like a Greek chorus, "Something powerful looms behind me. *Dark, huge, uncontrollable.*"

On May 19, 1998, I was continuing a routine business trip from Paramus, New Jersey, thru White Plains, New York and into Connecticut. I awakened in the hotel that morning "knowing" I would have a car accident. I desperately wanted to end my business trip right then but feared my company would fire me for going home too early. How crazy would I sound telling my boss, "Look, I just know I'm going to have a car accident today. I swear people are aiming for me! I need to get off the road!" Yet this is how I felt.

Muscling through my fears, I took the easiest route I could and woke up at a red light. I heard honking horns as the beeps of my alarm clock. Thinking I must have fallen asleep and stalled the car, I briefly chastised my laziness.

Then I saw the woman behind me flailing arms around her "Oh, my God!" looking face. Dimly, I recalled a crash—*a really loud crash*—and thinking *Oh, my God, someone really GOT it!*

I slowly realized that "someone" was *me*. She must have hit my car from behind. She seemed so far away, though. *So far away, and I'm so tired. Just woke up. Why can't my car become my bed again?*

We pulled our vehicles to the side of the road and tried to exchange insurance information. Only I could not figure out what "insurance information" was. After three or four botched attempts to produce my registration, I asked the woman to find what she wanted in my glove compartment. She removed a registration card and recorded my name and address.

I remember nothing of the drive home except passing through a tollbooth in Newark, New Jersey, thinking, "If I were smart, I'd pull over and go to a hospital, but I want my bed. I want my sheets." I could feel their cool chambray on my skin.

The next thing I knew, I was pulling into my parents' driveway in Bethlehem, Pennsylvania, trying not to vomit. I guess I decided to stop at their house because they lived closer to White Plains than I did.

I often passed through Bethlehem for dinner on return trips to my apartment near Philadelphia. This stop seemed ordinary enough to my parents. Since I had fainted in the past from hunger, they assumed my extreme nausea and dizziness meant I needed to eat. They insisted I join them out for dinner.

At the restaurant that night, I could not read the menu. The letters swam, so I asked my dad to order fish. Nauseous, I barely touched my plate.

On the way home, my mother suggested I pick out a movie at Blockbuster "to relax." I stood for twenty minutes, viewing both copies of *Much Ado about Nothing*. How could I decide which box to pick? Unaware of thousands of other titles, I grew so overwhelmed I needed to leave.

Outside, in the sweltering parking lot, I wanted to heave. I felt drunk and hung-over at the same time. Drunk, like: "Oh, no! I have the spins." Hung-over like: "I want to rip my stomach out as soon as I take the jack hammer out of my head."

I spent the night at my parents' house and slept for 16 hours—about 10 hours longer than I usually slept. I awoke in a stupor, called my parents at work, and they insisted I see a physician.

Heading south on the Pennsylvania Turnpike, I reached my doctor's office an hour later. He diagnosed me with a "moderate concussion" and ordered me to take a week off work. I laughed the whole way home, unable to articulate what seemed so funny.

Still nauseous, I needed to remind myself that red means "stop" and green means "go." Every time someone honked at me for pausing at a green light, I tried to control my laughter. Rarely, did I succeed. The world seemed gloriously funny as it spun around me. It never even occurred to me that I should not be driving.

I called a few of my friends, trying to ground myself with conversation. Enough was enough! I tired of feeling drunk, and the imaginary hangover grew more intense.

This did not feel like the times I'd been knocked out playing soccer or racquetball and had shaken off my confusion for a quick return to action. This time, I felt like I had cobwebs not only in my mouth, but in my entire brain.

My tongue felt tangled, caught inside itself; my brain, the attic in *Jane Eyre*—locked and howling. Whenever someone asked a question, I waded through cobwebs to find an answer. I could not understand how my head got so dusty when I was still there cleaning.

Every time I cleared a cobweb, a thicker one reappeared. My thoughts were suffocating in a dim and haunted brain.

I continued driving, despite needing tremendous willpower not to vomit after my journeys. Sometimes I forgot my destination. No matter. As long as I did not stop, I would not have to feel the car's motion continue in my body.

I dreaded the end of my drives. When I lay down on the bed, it slid away from the wall. The bookcases came at me like traffic. My stomach remembered every turn of the road and lurched again.

My body and brain replayed each trip forty or fifty times, long after I had parked the car. After driving to my parents' house for a visit—one hour away—I spent 48 hours prostrate on the gliding bed before I could drive home again. Curious and embarrassed, I told no one.

*   *   *

A week after my accident, I attempted to work from home. Looking at my laptop became an adventure. Each glance summoned a wave of vertigo that occasionally knocked me off the chair. After a few spills, I learned to hold one chair arm as I opened my customer database.

Dialing phone numbers made me laugh and then nearly unleashed a growing rage. I could not focus on one line at a time, so I kept misdialing numbers. I transposed area codes, calling one place and asking for a buyer at their other store. Sometimes I called the right person, apparently forgot, and then called again five minutes later. If they acted surprised and a little irritated, I took it personally.

Since I could not remember how to get to any of my clients' stores, I now only worked from home. Intending to take a quick lunch break from computer-induced vertigo, I went to the grocery store across the street from my apartment. When I saw the florescent glare off too-white floors, my eyes hurt. "Be fast," I thought, "You can do this." But fast, I was not.

Five times, I wandered by the same man offering samples of Italian sausage. I explained to him that I was vegetarian and did not eat pork. As I drifted through the store, his presence became familiar. I felt grateful for his repeated "hellos," because they grounded me when the room began to spin. He was like the starting line on a circular track, orienting me each time I passed.

After five laps, I had still not selected any food. "OK," I smiled at the man, "I'll buy some sausage." I, the starry-eyed vegetarian, bought a family pack.

"With the sausage I need spaghetti," I reasoned, "and some sauce." The sauce stumped me. I stood in front of all the brands and wanted to run. *Prego or Ragu?* It seemed monumental and confusing, even though I had always hated Prego. I eventually closed my eyes and grabbed a bottle. *Prego it was.*

When I arrived home, the time disturbed me. I had left my apartment shortly after 11 a.m. I bought nothing but pasta, Prego and those sausages. It was now after 1:00.

*   *   *

Sometime in mid-June, my dad arrived to drive me to my parents' home. Staying there made driving me to the next six doctors' appointments far less inconvenient for them.

Years later, I learned the *real* reason behind these mandatory three-day visits. My parents were terrified to leave me more than 36 hours alone in my apartment, but feared I might go mad without this last illusion of independence.

My business line rang, and I had a ten-minute conversation with a customer. When I hung up, my father asked me with whom I spoke. "Oh, I don't know," I said, "Some client or other." "Do you know which one?" he asked. "Of course I do," I lied.

When I tried to think about the conversation, I drew a total blank. After a bit more grilling from my father, I explained to him that my business conversations were confidential. "I really can't talk to you about my clients."

"Laura," he said, "You sell shoe trees to department stores! I can go in any of them and see your products on their shelves."

I did not want to admit how many cobwebs filled my brain. How could I fit insignificant facts into this fuzzy mess? I swept away some cobwebs for another excuse but found none.

"I'm hungry," I asserted. "Let's eat."

*   *   *

I was beginning to think I might have a real problem with my brain. I suddenly found myself between two rows of books with no idea where I was or how I had arrived.

Trying not to look as panicked as I felt, I searched the scene for anything recognizable. I checked my pockets: no car keys. I must have walked.

The only place with lots of books within walking distance of my apartment was the local library. I must have decided to get a book on tape to quell my boredom. Any attempts to read resulted in excruciating headaches and vertigo, but reading helped distract from constant nausea. Maybe I had thought a book on tape would do the trick without all those dizzy and painful side effects.

In any case, I was too flustered to select anything from those too long audio shelves. I left the library, trying to remember where I lived.

*   *   *

Six weeks of forgetting conversations with customers, misquoting prices, sleeping half the workday and showing few signs of imminent improvement forced me to go on Worker's Compensation.

May, June, July and August 1998 remain a blur of neurological, chiropractic, ophthalmologic and physical therapy appointments—all submitted to Worker's Compensation insurance.

I was not really getting any better; I had just learned what *not* to do:

- No reading
- No florescent lights
- No talking to more than one person at a time
- No phone calls over ten minutes
- No plucking eyebrows
- No lights on when I had a headache (most of the time!)
- No more than two 24-hour migraine pills/day
- No less than six migraine pills/week
- No days without a nap
- No driving more than three miles at a time
- No driving at night

- No watching videos without all the lights on
- No special effects
- No fans
- No prisms
- No large hand gestures
- No riding in the back seat
- No looking at oncoming headlights
- Never go anywhere without my sunglasses

By late August, my Worker's Comp insurance carrier began to grow impatient. From their location in Wisconsin (near my employer's headquarters), they assigned a Pennsylvania caseworker to accompany me on all major doctors' appointments.

I became a dollar figure, an expensive liability—maxing out the Temporary Total Disability (TTD) compensation level and accumulating medical bills disproportionately high to my rate of recovery.

They didn't care that I could not attend graduate school as planned, or that life as I knew it had ceased to exist. According to my caseworker, my insurance company wanted to get rid of me. Step one: an "Independent" Medical Evaluation (IME) with a doctor of their choice.

On September 16, 1998, the day before my first IME (ironically, the same day I would have started graduate school), I received the results of my EEG—a graphical recording of the electrical impulses of my brain. Surprised and not entirely relieved, I learned that an objective test shows signs of brain damage.

My "left temporal lobe" looked "moderately abnormal," and there was "asymmetrical activity" in my "occipital drivers." *(Left-brain function includes short-term memory, sequential reasoning, and decision-making. Occipital drivers control the eyes. "Asymmetrical activity" indicated that my eyes did not always work together.)*

This report would surely seal the IME, but it also meant that my "imaginary" injury was real. I went for a walk to digest the news.

Remembering a giant cave-like painting of two jackals I had seen in my neurologist, Dr. Jackel's, office, I suddenly felt eyes upon me. I looked up in time to see a Doberman running across the lawn at me.

At first, I assumed there was a fence. I looked again: no fence. "Surely," I thought, "They must have one of those invisible electronic fences." I wanted to run, but then I remembered my recurring dream. The dog reached the edge of the lawn and started to cross the street.

My panic turned to laughter. "So this is it! I get the EEG in time for the IME, but I don't make it to the IME because a Doberman devours my butt." Just then, the owner called her dog off, and I wandered home in my usual daze. Apparently, brain injury works wonders for non-attachment.

*   *   *

Before my car accident, I spent my time meeting sales quotas, traveling, and counting down the days to graduate school. My shift into a life with TBI seemed no less dramatic or implausible than Dorothy's move from Kansas into Munchkin Land.

Like Dorothy, I knew I could not return the way I had arrived. Like Dorothy, I eventually found my way "back home," but I took the Technicolor journey with me. I wrote this book to help others do so, too.

Glinda

What person suffering from chronic pain or disability has not wished for a magic wand to take it all away? In the strange land of TBI, who would not smile with relief at the appearance of a Glinda?

Alas, the Good Witch of the North will not emerge from a pink bubble to whisk you back to health. Nonetheless, some people *can* help you in surprising and unusual ways.

This chapter suggests ways to find the Glinda's along your journey. Be prepared to work, though. Even in *The Wizard of Oz*, Glinda prefers to help Dorothy help herself.

1. *Contact organizations and support groups.*

Most hospitals have a TBI advocacy group that will put you in touch with people in similar situations. Brain injury can feel very isolating because you and other people cannot "see" the damage.

Sometimes you might even wonder if your injury is real. Interacting with someone who understands how it feels to have a brain injury will help ease your loneliness and self-doubt.

You can also interact with survivors online by joining an international TBI-Survivor email group at *www.braininjurychat.org*. Many people think of the other group members as "family."

If you have a different injury or illness, look for support from hospital and online groups for people in your situation.

I wish I had known about brain injury organizations in the early stage of my recovery. Until I encountered other survivors, I felt like a freak. I learned later that many people with brain injuries suffer from oversensitivity, visual problems, and difficulty making decisions.

I was not, as my insurance company claimed, "a medical mystery." Just knowing that someone else shared the same struggles relieved a great deal of anxiety.

If you have not already done so, contact a state or national brain injury organization. Your doctor may not have much experience with TBI, but these groups exist to educate and assist people with neurological problems ranging from concussion to severe TBI.

In addition to explaining your symptoms within a larger TBI context, these organizations can sometimes recommend physicians and attorneys in your region:

- Brain Injury Association of America:
  800-444-6443 or *www.biausa.org*
- Brain Injury Resource Center:
  www.headinjury.com This organization offers tons of resources, including ways to get funding for education or self-employment.
- National Resource Center for Traumatic Brain Injury:
  www.neuro.pmr.vcu.edu
- Jamaica Hospital Medical Center:
  www.tbihelp.org
  This site emphasizes Caregiver Resources, too.

You might also want to consider other organizations that can help. I suffered mainly from visual dysfunction. When I had recovered enough to look for limited part-time work, I contacted my state's Society for the Blind and Visually Impaired. They reviewed my medical records, vocational goals and job experience in order to find possible career matches.

State and federally funded, the Society for the Blind and Visually Impaired could recommend and pay for a larger monitor and any software to aid computer usage.

Best of all, the organization exists to serve people with no or very impaired vision. I felt truly understood for the first time not by a neurologist, but by a (blind) vocational rehabilitation specialist. **Depending on your symptoms, you may find more empathy and help from a non-brain injury organization:**

- Fibromyalgia Network, a membership program (\$28/year) for people with Fibromyalgia and Chronic Fatigue Syndrome, "aim(s) to educate and assist patients with ad-free, patient-focused information that they can put to use today."
  http://www.fmnetnews.com/
- The National Fibromyalgia Association provides links to support groups across the nation:
  http://www.fmaware.org/site/PageServer
- Lyme Disease Association, Inc. (LDA), a non-profit organization, offers general information, doctor referrals, resources and links to support groups. Their LymeAid 4 Kids program also offers money to families with uninsured, Lyme infected children.
  http://www.lymediseaseassociation.org/
- Centers for Disease Control and Prevention (CDC) offer information on how to select a Chronic Fatigue Syndrome support group, along with links to support groups in and outside the United States:
  http://www.cdc.gov
- *http://www.migrainepage.com/* offers a place for migraine sufferers to post journal entries, artwork, articles and online chat about their experiences with other people who get migraines or cluster headaches.
- *http://www.braintrust.org/* offers peer-led online support groups for people with brain cancer, including tumor-specific groups.
- The Family Caregiver Alliance offers an online support group for family and other caregivers of people with Alzheimer's, brain injury, stroke or other chronic and debilitating health issues:
  www.caregiver.org.

- *www.CarePages.com* provides a virtual meeting place on the web, so that geographically distanced family members can stay updated, view photos, and offer support. This saves time and energy when caregivers or survivors want to reach out but can't feasibly contact everyone via phone or email. The site also offers articles and resources organized by ailment.

2. Have a neuropsychological evaluation.

In the legal arena, a neuropsychological evaluation can demonstrate brain damage that fails to register on tests like Magnetic Resonance Imaging (MRI) or CAT scan.

(Claustrophobics, beware of the MRI experience. You lie strapped down in a suffocating tube of clanging echoes for what seems like hours, and the test rarely confirms mild or moderate TBI. Instead, you receive a "normal" evaluation, which seems to refute your claim.)

Most neuropsychologists include a malingering test, in order to rule out the possibility of faking or exaggeration. These experts compare your performance in various areas with anticipated performance based on your education, previous test scores (if available) and former occupation. They will also compare your results with those of other people suffering similar brain damage.

The information gleaned from a neuropsychological evaluation can provide important clues to your recovery. Ideally, therapists tailor your recovery program to correct the specific problems you exhibit. Cognitive rehabilitation therapy helps to improve short-term memory and concentration ability. Your rehab specialist can also give you ideas for coping with current and lasting impairments.

If your brain damage becomes extremely noticeable and/or does not improve in a month, you might want to begin pushing for a neuropsychological evaluation.

My primary care physician thought the four-to-eight hour test would be "too traumatic" for me and discouraged me from taking one. On his recommendation, my neurologist did not order a test until three months after my TBI.

The trauma hospital was so backlogged that my first neuropsychological evaluation occurred on November 4, 1998—almost six months after the accident. Even so, my IQ remained 47 points below pre-injury test levels.

Unfortunately, my high school had destroyed most of my records when I turned 25 (three days after the accident). Without a document to prove my old IQ, few medical personnel took the 47-point drop as seriously as I did.

In May 2000, a different neuropsychologist performed a second evaluation. In the year and a half since my first test, my IQ had risen twenty points. Since it was clear I remained significantly impaired, the jump supported how injured I must have been on May 19, 1998.

Throughout my recovery, I participated in two extensive malingering tests, both of which indicated "a malingering probability of zero." Nevertheless, insurance company "hired guns" (physicians selected to write reports that indicated I was faking) held the six-month testing delay against me. They argued that if my symptoms had been as severe as I claimed, I would have taken the neuropsych exam immediately.

Optimism about recovery is wonderful: it's true, such expensive, formal testing just might prove unnecessary. Unfortunately, insurance restrictions and lawsuits encourage one to establish "evidence" early on. A supportive neuropsych evaluation might also make doctors take your complaints more seriously.

3. Consult a behavioral optometrist.

A behavioral or neuro-optometrist specializes in connections among mind, body, and vision. Many seemingly non-visual problems have their root cause in visual dysfunction.

According to the Neuro-Optometric Rehabilitation Association (NORA), a majority of people with neurological issues suffer from visual impairment. If you have any of the following symptoms, you may benefit from visual therapy or prism lenses:

- Concentration problems
- Double vision
- Headaches
- Difficulty reading
- Balance disorders
- Clumsiness
- Eyestrain
- Intolerance of flickering lights
- Intolerance to varied backgrounds
- Panic attacks
- Easily becoming overwhelmed
- Vertigo

Traditional doctors could not explain or cure my migraine-like headaches. I eventually worked with two behavioral optometrists, and my headaches disappeared. When selecting a visual therapist, try to find one who has worked with TBI or stroke patients, as treatment techniques can vary widely.

Both of my behavioral optometrists gave me home vision exercises (i.e. crawling, balancing on one foot, or following my moving thumb with my eyes but not my head). However, their in-office approaches could not have been more different.

My Seattle, Washington doctor performed CranioSacral therapy (see Hint #4) on me while I moved my eyes in uncomfortable positions. An herbalist renowned for improving vision with nutritional supplements, he also prescribed these liberally (see Hint #25).

By contrast, my Evanston, Illinois doctor listed six exercises for me to do per session. Progressively more difficult, the exercises involved anything from hopping on a trampoline to walking with glasses that made the floor look crooked. His assistants would observe and correct me until I "graduated" to the next level.

Whereas my Seattle doctor relieved headaches with herbs and tissue manipulation, my Evanston doctor used a system of colored lights to cure nausea and vertigo. I spent 16 months with each doctor.

You can enter your location on the NORA website in order to find a behavioral optometrist near you: *www.nora.cc*; or, phone: 866-2CBETTER.

In Appendix 1: "Glinda's Secrets," Dr. William Padula shares more technical information about the field of neuro-optometric rehabilitation.

4. Try CranioSacral therapy.

My neurologist had prescribed trigger point injections of lidocaine to ease neck spasms. With the intent of eventually causing those muscles to relax, the doctor induced sixteen or more rapid spasms in each of my trigger points. The needles left dark bruises, and I felt sick to my stomach from the pain. I could not turn my head or lift my arms for several days after each session.

Because trigger point injections are expensive, my insurance company suspected me of trying to avoid—much cheaper but more frequent—physical therapy massages in order to have this "quick and easy" treatment. I *was* trying to streamline my treatment options, but not because I found trigger point injections "quick" or "easy" compared to a massage!

The injections happened once monthly, and after work my parents drove me a silent one hour to an incandescently lit and relaxing office; the physical therapy massages required my taking a twenty-minute to one-hour handicapped van ride three times per week to a hospital with glaring florescent lights.

The lurching, fluorescently lit van with people yelling nonsense syllables made me incredibly nauseous. Apparently, not just me: on my last van ride, another passenger puked on my canvas shoe!

When the insurance company had their caseworker observe one of my trigger point sessions, she turned away after the first ten twitches, unable to stomach my revolting display of angry muscles.

Dreading the trigger point injections almost as much as my original symptoms, I searched for other options. I experienced more immediate and lasting relief through weekly CranioSacral treatments.

With its non-invasive touch, CranioSacral Therapy (CST) often produces dramatic results in the management of chronic neck and back pain, migraine headaches, and recovery from TBI. Available from massage and physical therapists and my behavioral optometrist, CST relaxed my system instead of re-traumatizing it.

If you have symptoms that have not responded to traditional medicine, you might want to investigate CST.

John Upledger, an osteopathic physician and Professor of Biomechanics at University of Michigan, developed CST after extensive scientific research. According to the Upledger Institute:

> *"CST is a gentle, hands-on method of evaluating and enhancing the functioning of . . . the craniosacral system—comprised of the membranes and cerebrospinal fluid that surround and protect the brain and spinal cord . . . . Using a soft touch . . . , practitioners release restrictions*

in the craniosacral system to improve the functioning of the central nervous system."

Developed for neurological use, CST also works on soft connective tissue and the lymphatic system. It is usually considered an "alternative treatment"; however, your practitioner may be able to bill CST under the heading of a more traditional umbrella like massage or physical therapy.

On the Upledger Institute's website, you can learn more about CST, as well as locate a practitioner near you: *www.upledger.com.*

5. *Get evaluated for Lyme Disease.*

When an expert in vertigo ordered my first test for Lyme Disease, I felt betrayed. True, I lived and hiked near one of the highest populations of Lyme diseased patients, but *come on*! I functioned perfectly fine until I hit my head on May 19, 1998. I viewed the Lyme test as yet another attempt by Worker's Comp to claim my symptoms arose from another cause than TBI.

The physician ordered about 20 blood tests in all, including the one for Lyme. I wondered if I had any blood left when they finished taking the final vial. Oddly enough, the results of my Lyme titer disappeared en route from the lab. Twice.

Mystified and apologetic for sending me to the fluorescent hospital for yet another Lyme test, the physician agreed that given their timing it was most unlikely my symptoms stemmed from Lyme Disease. Privately, I wondered how this "expert" could ever have even considered such a possibility.

Despite living in a region of Pennsylvania with a huge population of deer known to carry ticks infected with the *Borrelia burgdorferi* spirochete, the agent of Lyme Disease, I did not consider this infection in the same league as say, head trauma. I knew about the characteristic "bulls-eye" rash around a tick bite, but I had never seen such a rash. I had heard that one side of one's face could droop but that antibiotics would fix even that problem within a couple weeks.

My parents' dog caught Lyme: she limped and felt tired for a few days before a veterinarian found the problem and prescribed antibiotics. My nephew caught Lyme when he was two, and again, a course of antibiotics seemed to do the trick.

True, a friend of mine nearly died from heart inflammation caused by the bacteria, but again, antibiotics cured the problem after diagnosis. The heart part seemed scary, but from everything I knew about Lyme Disease, it shared nothing in common with long-term neurological symptoms. In my opinion, it was an infection like strep throat: easily treated and quickly resolved.

For five years, I thought little more of Lyme Disease, particularly after I moved to the arid southwest, which seemed far removed from the overpopulated deer runs of Pennsylvania.

In October 2004, my husband Stephen and I had just bought a car that decided to breakdown at every possible opportunity. One day, the engine light came on, and Stephen lifted the hood to evaluate the problem. Nothing seemed unusual, so he bent closer, leaning over the engine in a loose fitting Edgar Allen Poe T-shirt.

Unable to locate the problem, we resigned ourselves to another trip to the mechanic, who told us he had found a large field mouse nest near the engine. The nights had recently turned cool, and field mice liked a toasty engine to keep them warm. The mechanic blew out the mouse nest, and we gave no more thought to the incident.

About a week or so later, Stephen developed an odd rash underneath one armpit. It seemed to radiate out from a central point of irritation, and it looked patchy. It healed in the center first, yet lingered for weeks. Even though he had used the same type of deodorant for years and only had a rash in one armpit, we assumed he had developed an allergy to his deodorant. Eventually the rash disappeared, and we thought no more of it.

Around the same time, Stephen caught the flu. He felt like hell, and he lost his voice for three weeks. He became extremely light sensitive, and his monitor suddenly seemed unbearably blurry. We shared a tiny room together, but I never caught anything.

In retrospect, we should have taken him to the doctor, but Stephen is a veteran, and the nearest facility was over an hour away. The thought of driving through rain in our car with a leaky roof, dying differential, bad tires and malfunctioning headlights encouraged us to let him recover at home.

I researched illnesses noted for skin rashes: chicken pox, shingles. Nothing seemed to fit. My intuition screamed "Lyme Disease," but I rationally dismissed it as an "East Coast thing." I never even looked at photos of the bullseye rash, because I did not want to waste my time on impossibilities.

Eventually, the flu symptoms disappeared and his voice returned, but over the next few months, Stephen continued to complain about his vision. Two optometrists evaluated him, and his prescription had changed so little that it did not explain the blurriness. He bought a new monitor and new glasses: still blurry.

Stephen became increasingly irritable and short-tempered. Little things that never used to bother him suddenly caused a huge reaction:

- The sun was too bright
- The radio too loud
- The breeze on his skin too much
- The light on his headset too blue
- The neighbors too disrespectful
- And his head hurt *all* the time.

About the time he caught the "flu," Stephen had started talking in opposites. If he meant to say, "Let's go there tomorrow," he would actually say, "Let's go there yesterday."

At first, we laughed, but then it began happening more frequently. We suffered many a misunderstanding because in Stephen's mind, he said one thing, but what he verbalized was frequently the exact opposite of what he intended. We thought either I was going deaf or Stephen was going crazy.

My sister is a speech pathologist, and she had never heard of such a specific speech aberration. Nor had my neurologist aunt and uncle. Since no one had any answers, and it seemed harmless enough, I simply took to "translating" whatever Stephen said.

This usually worked unless he happened to say something correctly. Then he wondered why I had the audacity to do the exact opposite of what we had agreed! This talking in opposite continued for years.

We decided Stephen needed a change of pace, so we moved to Lake Tahoe. Stephen had lived at 8,400 feet before with no altitude sickness, but when we arrived in Nevada, he could barely breathe. His chest hurt, and he grew so tired I often half-dragged him to bed.

The V.A. Medical Center had a three-month wait for appointments, and Stephen did not feel well enough to drive an hour to the emergency room. I bought him liquid oxygen, and he started feeling better. I encouraged him to sit in the sun, and it seemed to do him good.

As the weather warmed, he started taking photographs, and the new pursuit further lifted his health and spirits. (You can view and purchase Stephen's photos on *www.stephenbrunophotography.com*). Creativity does wonders for chronic ailments!

After an EKG and standard blood tests, Stephen received a clean bill of health from the V.A. We thought it must have been the altitude and cold weather after all, and as a precaution moved somewhere lower.

As the weather grew cold again, Stephen became increasingly irritable. "Nothing works for me anymore!" he complained of his monitor, our apartment, the squeaky noise in our new car, light between the window blinds, food smells, scented soap, his formerly cherished hamburgers.

I barely recognized the laid-back man I had married:

- His hands shook all the time
- His chest felt tender
- He felt things "crawling around in his chest"
- He had excruciating headaches every day
- Sometimes, he could not even get out of bed
- His symptoms seemed to peak every fourth week

I brought him meals and started giving him Oil of Oregano as a general immune system tonic. Stephen improved.

Until I ran out of Oil of Oregano—which happens to be a natural, but extremely potent antibiotic. Within days:

- One side of his face felt numb
- His chest hurt like a heart attack
- His right knee ached so he could barely walk
- His eyes twitched
- Skin burned
- And his head felt more explosive than usual.

I insisted he go to a doctor. I could not stop thinking and talking about Lyme Disease, so I finally looked up the symptoms on the internet. Stephen had every listed symptom, including a propensity to talk in opposites.

Then my jaw dropped: the ticks carrying *Borrelia burgdorferi* also feast on field mice! Once I remembered the weird rash, we insisted the doctors give him antibiotics. Stephen improved dramatically.

Until his prescription ended.

Thus began a cycle in which his symptoms all but disappeared as long as Stephen remained on some form of potent antibiotic. No infection appeared in countless blood tests, and all other tests returned normal as well. Yet, any move off antibiotics resulted in an imminent trip to the ER with chest pain, a meningitis scare, rapidly progressing skin rash, or headaches so severe he could not concentrate.

After three months, the V.A. refused to give Stephen any more antibiotics, saying they could not justify the expense or risk to his health.

I put him back on Oil of Oregano, figuring it could not hurt. Again, Stephen improved. I could tell by his behavior if he had taken a dose within a few hours or was overdue. I found someone at the local co-op who suffered from a confirmed case of Lyme Disease. His story and symptoms sounded strikingly like Stephen's. This man highly recommended a supplement called **Prima Una de Gato**. Combined with **Oil of Oregano** and **Teasel Root**, it has worked wonders.

In November 2006, one of Stephen's doctors finally agreed to a specialized test offered by the Bowen Group. This QRiBb test actually photographs the spirochetes (Lyme bacteria) in someone's blood. Sure enough, Stephen was still in the mid-high category of infection.

His doctor immediately prescribed antibiotics and encouraged me to continue the herbal protocol. In his words, Stephen was "lucky to be alive" given his earlier meningitis symptoms and the V.A.'s refusal to medicate him. As long as he continues his doses, Stephen shows few of his previous symptoms. If he goes without their immune-boosting effects, his symptoms begin to return, but over time, we have high hopes for a full recovery.

Lyme Disease can be difficult to diagnose and even more difficult to treat. The spirochete form of *Borrelia burgdorferi* allows the bacteria to burrow through cells and evade detection by both blood tests and the host's immune system. They can form cysts and lie dormant for years, breaking out when the immune system becomes impaired through stress, trauma or another illness.

Some doctors consider Lyme Disease the #1 vector-borne illness in the United States. Related to syphilis, the Lyme spirochete is sometimes called, "the new great imitator" because it wreaks havoc in the same unpredictable and multiple ways that syphilis can.

With ties to M.S., ALS (Lou Gehrig's Disease), arthritis, Fibromyalgia, stroke, vision problems, and Chronic Fatigue Syndrome, Lyme Disease is an under-reported and often misdiagnosed illness. It turns out my vertigo expert had been wise to examine Lyme as a possibility!

Because of its difficult detection, widespread, "non-specific" symptoms, and the potential expense of long-term treatment, Lyme Disease has become one of the most controversial topics among medical professionals and insurance companies. People speak of "Lyme Literate" doctors as either saviors or quacks.

Accurate testing remains a challenge, though labs like Igenex and Bowen seem to detect more positive results than many other labs do. In short, Lyme might have nothing to do with any of your symptoms, and even if it does, that fact might not reveal itself in an objective test. Many Lyme Literate doctors diagnose by symptoms and positive response to antibiotics rather than relying solely on a frequently unreliable blood test.

Having experienced my own TBI and then observed my husband's struggles with similar symptoms, I observed first hand that the effectiveness of any treatment depends on the underlying cause of symptoms. Lavender essential oil, Advil, and ice packs do not stop Stephen's headaches or calm his eyes, whereas Oil of Oregano or an antibiotic do. Conversely, improving my own immune system kept me from getting sick, but did nothing to improve my migraines.

Proper diagnosis neither guarantees nor eliminates the possibility of recovery. But it *can* help you to aim treatment efforts in the right direction.

6. *Choose your lawyer carefully.*

Do not settle for anyone other than an expert in his or her field. Brain injury litigation can become extremely complicated—especially if you have unusual symptoms or did not immediately recognize the severity of your injury.

Your lawyer must be able to explain your problems in understandable terms and prove a direct connection between the accident and your injuries. If the attorney does not offer prior successful experience with TBI cases, you probably want to search elsewhere.

My Workers' Comp attorney had never worked a brain injury case before mine; however, he offered 25 years experience in Workers' Comp litigation. He knew the laws inside and out, and his expertise earned me a settlement.

He constantly refrained, "Simple wins. We have to boil this complicated case into its most simple components. Then it will not only be believable: it will become the only logical explanation."

He distilled a seven-inch stack of medical, school and employment records into a basic formula: as demonstrated by work and academic achievements, Laura functioned well before her accident; she damaged her brain in the accident, and she could no longer function after the accident; therefore, the accident and TBI caused her inability to function. Whatever complexities the defense raised, my attorney repeated this easy explanation. His tactic worked.

My personal injury lawyer, on the other hand, initially had no knowledge of brain injury and less overall experience. Successful with straightforward cases, he grew fascinated by all the angles and innuendos of my suffering.

In his determination to show the jury every devastating facet of this life-changing injury, he forgot to emphasize basic connections among accident, injury, and pain and suffering. He also opted for an economist instead of an accident reconstructionist or biomechanical engineer.

The defense could afford at least five lawyers working against my one. Consequently, the defense found loopholes—like excluding medical records from evidence—while my lawyer drowned in details.

Because of the pervasive effects on survivor's lives, most law firms view TBI cases as opportunities for multi-million dollar settlements. Ironically, the fact that TBI touches so much of a person's life makes much of that person's life open to discussion. With so many factors involved, a jury can more easily find "Reasonable Doubts."

If a jury accepts the injury, then they will generally award enormous compensation. If a lawyer fails to explain the connections among accident, injury and symptoms, then the victim often walks away with nothing.

The "all or nothing" character of TBI claims increases the importance of having an experienced attorney on your side.

The American Bar Association has approved a free referral service to find high profile lawyers in your area, including ones specializing in traumatic brain injury:

> **866-LAW4USA or** *www.getareferral.com*. Some hospitals and support groups will also offer their suggestions.

Note: *Location matters*! Especially if you found yourself injured in a car accident or on the job—or in my case, both. I had three states involved: Pennsylvania (where I lived), New York (where the accident took place) and Wisconsin (my company's headquarters). Even if it seems like too much trouble to research differing state laws, you could save yourself years of agony and thousands to millions of dollars by choosing the right jurisdiction. I include my story as an example:

In 1998, a law student erroneously told me that no lawyer would take my Worker's Compensation case without a personal injury suit attached to it. When Worker's Comp started pulling the purse strings on treatment, I visited an attorney friend of a friend who handled both Worker's Compensation and personal injury cases—*in Pennsylvania*. I signed paperwork with him to the effect that if I needed representation from him, I would have it. I hoped I would never need him, and thought no more of lawsuits.

One day, a lawyer from New York called to say he had taken over my personal injury claim. He explained that because the accident had occurred in New York, I needed a New York attorney and that the Pennsylvania lawyer had transferred all the paperwork to his firm. While the pre-injury "me" would have resisted this turn of affairs—I did not even get to select my own attorney—the brain-injured "me" said, "Fine, I have a really bad headache, and I probably won't remember the details anyway."

It turns out, those details were important. The Pennsylvania attorney had turned my entire case (both Worker's Compensation and personal injury) over to this New York firm; however, the New York firm could not handle a Worker's Compensation claim from Pennsylvania *or* Wisconsin! My New York and Pennsylvania attorneys told me I needed a Wisconsin attorney for Worker's Compensation, which "absolutely fell under Wisconsin's jurisdiction" even though I lived in Pennsylvania.

Guess what? When my sister married a Pennsylvania Workers Compensation attorney, I learned that this, too, was erroneous advice. I could have demanded a Pennsylvania jurisdiction—and should have, because (in 1998 anyway) Pennsylvania laws "favor the victim, whereas

Wisconsin favors the insurance companies." Because my job injury became a Wisconsin claim, the burden of proof shifted to me.

My insurance company, could (and did) shop me around to "Independent" Medical Examiners until they could find someone to state I had faked my symptoms. As soon as they had that report, they could legally cut off all treatment approval, disability checks and reimbursement—even though their own doctor's test showed a "malingering probability of zero." I then needed to spend months fighting to get those expenses and salary substitutes reimbursed. In Pennsylvania, they could not have stopped my benefits without first winning in court.

When your brain stops working, the last thing you want to do is research your rights, but it can make a huge difference in the funds you receive for treatment. Time and money matter in the course of your recovery. If you can't keep track of the complexities, find someone who can—a friend, family member, social worker, church member, or counselor. Keep asking for what you need. *Someone* will listen and come through for you!

Ruby Slippers and the
Wicked Witch of the West

When the Wicked Witch finds herself dispossessed of the Ruby Slippers, she rages, "I'm the only one who knows how to use them!" Intimidated, Dorothy would relinquish all their power, just to placate the witch.

Fortunately, Glinda provides wisdom and encouragement when Dorothy feels most vulnerable: "They must be very powerful, or she wouldn't want them so badly."

You hold within you the key to your true healing. Just as the Ruby Slippers click Dorothy home, this key can unlock wellness. You probably have some sense of what real healing would involve. This key glitters and shines like the Ruby Slippers, even though you do not—cannot—understand it.

As soon as you try to grasp the key, *ego*—your resident Wicked Witch—attempts to hide the lock. Ego recognizes what you do not: the latent power you hold in your possession. If you learn how to use your key to healing, then ego will lose control. Like the Wicked Witch, your ego will do anything for power.

Yet this key belongs to you—to the Essence of you. Just as Ruby Slippers magically appear on Dorothy's feet, so the key rightfully belongs to your highest Self. You cannot give it away, no matter how much your ego threatens and insults you.

Before your injury, you probably never imagined such a thing's existence. Dorothy certainly never hears of Ruby Slippers until she needs them. The slippers cling to her feet long before they gain her entrance to the Emerald City, but she remains unaware of their potential until the proper time.

The potential for true healing remains within you, just as Dorothy could have clicked her heels home anytime in Oz. If you embrace this potential, you will find yourself more "alive"—and perhaps even healthier—than you were before your brain went haywire.

The suggestions in this chapter will help you overcome your inner Wicked Witch.

7. *Forgive yourself for taking so long to recover.*

The Brain—is wider than the Sky—
For—put them side by side—
The one the other will contain
With ease—and You—beside—

The Brain is deeper than the sea—
For—hold them—Blue to Blue—
The one the other will absorb—
As Sponges—Buckets—do—

The Brain is just the weight of God—
For—Heft them—Pound for Pound—
And they will differ—if they do—
As Syllable from Sound—

Emily Dickinson #632

One blow to the brain changes an entire lifetime of acquired skills and coping mechanisms. How old were you when you hit your head? It took you that many years to become who you were pre-injury. Your brain works day and night to repair itself, but it has millions of neuro-pathways to reconnect.

If the slow timeframe still troubles you, then make an honest assessment of your attitude and willingness to recover. If you consistently do everything in your power to heal, then stop judging yourself. If you recognize areas that impede your progress, then focus on resolving those issues. Feeling guilty will not get you well. Commitment and truth will.

Whether diagnosed with a concussion, head trauma, traumatic brain injury, stroke or brain cancer, you suffered physical damage to your brain. If you have Fibromyalgia, Chronic Fatigue Syndrome, or MS, the cognitive problems you experience are common. And real.

Emotional issues might play a role in your recovery, but you are not "crazy," "weak," "hysterical" or "mentally ill." You have brain damage, and you need to heal. How can you heal if you will not admit that you need healing?

I personally found it easier to doubt myself than to accept the vulnerability of my physical brain. I did not want to believe my sense of self depended so much upon biochemistry and nerve impulses. Until I recognized my limitations, I continued to push myself too hard.

Gently accepting the physical problems allowed me to relax without judgment. The rest and relaxation, in turn, allowed me to heal.

Remember that the apparent force of whatever hit your head does not necessarily indicate how severely you were injured. Factors like the impact's precise location, the cumulative effect of earlier TBI's, your age, and how many times your brain bounced inside your skull, can all influence recovery. You do not even need to hit your head on something external to sustain TBI. Whiplash, like Shaken Baby Syndrome, can sometimes kill.

Moreover, the actual force that hit your head may have been stronger than anybody calculated.

For example, after my accident, I had only looked at the damage to my own car, which seemed minor. I noticed a few scrapes on my rubber bumper, but nothing else. Dazed and nauseated, I did not waste my energy looking at the car that hit mine.

Because the woman's insurance company never volunteered information to suggest otherwise, I assumed I had survived a very minor accident with major complications. Doctors, Workers' Comp, employers and some family members treated me as a mysteriously sensitive and perhaps hysterical young woman. Even I wondered how I could have sustained such a life altering injury from a little bump.

In court, I finally learned the answer: my bumper was streaked across the hood of the other woman's car. She had not tapped me at a red light; she had slammed on her brakes so hard that her car dove under my car and threw it forward. The scrapes from my bumper exactly matched the black marks on her white car.

I can only imagine how different my TBI experience would have been had I known what really happened.

Would Workers' Comp have tried so hard to terminate my case? Probably. Would the other woman—a fastidiously dressed Bloomingdale's shopper—still have insisted the marks came from "a botched paint job in '95"? Probably, although she might have felt pressured to produce those records.

Would a jury have found my accident so difficult to believe? Maybe not.

I will never know, because my lawyer did not notice the marks until I pointed them out to him midway through trial. He had found the woman's evasive answers puzzling, but he worked my case as though I were "an eggshell victim," i.e. so delicate in my pre-injury state that it only took a tap to crack me.

The biggest difference I *can* know is how much guilt and self-doubt an accurate account of the accident would have spared me. To avoid senseless anger, I view the long held secret as an unusual twist of fate. I only share it with you to show that sometimes situations are not as they seem.

Go easy on yourself. In a world of insurance battles, legal nightmares and uncertain prognoses, someone has to.

8. *Recognize parts that needed to change.*

Without telling yourself that you "deserved" your injury or illness, take an honest look at your earlier attitudes, behaviors and expectations. Were you a kind person? A perfectionist? A workaholic? What did you value most? Least? What was your biggest regret before your health declined?

How have your answers to such questions changed as you developed chronic health problems? Since you cannot—at least for the moment—be the person you once were, take this opportunity to consider "how" and "whom" you *want* to be.

If you breezed through life, impatient with people who did not meet your expectations, maybe you now recognize the struggles of less gifted people. Think of how good it feels when someone accepts you as you are. You can become a tolerant person while you recover. Why not maintain that kindness when you're well?

Sometimes we know exactly what needs to change: a job, an unhappy marriage, an addiction. Other times, we might just sense a call to be a "better" or more authentic person. Many people with chronic health problems wrestle with judgments and perfectionism. Do your dreams conflict with your ideas of right and wrong? Of what's "professional?" Examine your options. You might find your current situation more of an opportunity to change than a permanent restriction.

9. *Draw upon what you already know.*

Your brain injury or illness probably initiated a bit of an identity crisis. I know mine did.

I remember waking up the next morning and wondering who this person was inside my head. She seemed vaguely familiar, but younger. Since I had spent that first night at my parents' house, I awoke in my old high school bed. At first, I actually thought I had wandered back through time.

Thought processes I had honed over many years suddenly seemed embryonic. I felt their potential, but they were definitely not accessible. I remembered this feeling.

It was the same feeling I had had in high school when I first discovered Plato and Descartes. I sensed something I might one day grasp, but it remained intangible—just outside articulation. My mind felt like my hand hanging out the window of a car and playing with the breeze. Exhilarated. Empty. Rising and falling on waves of air. Feeling the force, but grasping nothing.

As this state of mind appeared to take up permanent residence, I grew frustrated. A flashback to youth was one thing; having to start over quite another. I had already trained my mind in high school, college and graduate school. Why did I need to go through all that work again just to recognize myself? It seemed unfair, and I was angry.

Had I realized then that I would have to go much farther back—to the earliest stages of learning how to crawl—I would have revolted. Against what, I don't know, but I did not like this having to relearn.

It became clear that I could not force memories and thought patterns to reconnect through synapses. It would take a step-by-step process to reconstruct my brain. The hardest part for me was accepting that I could not find a short cut.

Once I acknowledged that I could find no other way, I recognized an overlooked advantage: I had already learned everything I needed to relearn. If I knew the goal and broke it down into components, then I ought to be able to arrive at it again. Once I humbled myself to practice crawling and to relearn critical thinking, I could focus on the task instead of on my wounded pride. I would devise my own curriculum. Like a child repeating grades, I had some idea what to expect.

I also had another advantage. I had not lost *all* my memories or skills. Experience and maturity gave me an edge, because I could use analogies for each new test. I knew what it felt like to score that soccer goal after weeks and weeks of shooting practice. I knew the satisfaction of completing a Masters Thesis after months of tedious research. In both cases, the build-up had seemed excessively long and frustrating, but in the end, I recognized its necessity.

Why should my recovery be any different? I wished it would be different—easier—but I had faced other challenges and triumphed. The greater the challenge, the greater the sense of achievement: I could do this.

When having to relearn the basics, remember what you already know. Just because parts of you changed does not mean you need to become an entirely different person. In renovating the dilapidated you, make strategic use of old materials. If you played sports before your TBI, then set up a "practice" regimen for yourself.

If you painted, think of your recovery as a work of art. A painting takes time to develop, and you might need to retouch several times before you get it right.

If you loved cooking, imagine your recovery as a banquet, for which you have just begun reading recipes.

Whatever your passion, whatever your insider knowledge—use to your advantage. Give yourself a context within which to work, so that you can recognize your progress.

10. *Follow your intuition.*

Has something been nagging you for a long time? Do you find yourself saying after the fact, "I *knew* that would happen!"? Do you often fight between rational thought and a strange, but persistent hunch?

Trust your hunches. People with neurological problems need whatever mental edge they can get. While compensating for cognitive damage, many people develop incredible intuitive capacities.

Throughout the course of my recovery, intuition led me to explore treatments and life choices that some physicians and family members considered suspect. Despite their advice, I learned to trust my intuitions.

Whenever I followed these internal promptings, I stumbled upon the right health care provider at the right time. On the second visit with one such doctor, my 16-month long migraine disappeared!

Although some people seem naturally more intuitive than others intuition is actually a skill that you can cultivate. As with any learned behavior, the more you practice, the better you will become. All it takes is awareness and an open mind.

Next time you need to make a decision, stop for a moment and pay attention to your body. How does it feel? Notice any lurches in your stomach when you consider certain options. Does one thought make your stomach tense, while the other gives you a sense of lightness inside? Where do you think the expression "gut feeling" comes from?

Now, notice other parts of your body. How's your breathing? Does your chest feel tight or free? Do you experience intense pain anywhere whenever you imagine yourself taking a particular course of action? If you were deciding something strictly based on how your body responds, what would you decide?

Listen to your body, especially when it screams for your attention.

Gut or visceral feelings form only one facet of intuition. Our emotions also speak to us, particularly fear and anxiety. Next time you are in a relaxed state, experiment with certain thoughts. Notice if your mind suddenly shifts into hyper-alert or panic mode. What were you thinking right before that happened?

Pay attention to any patterns. If something continually makes you cringe, then your intuition may be telling you to avoid that something or at least to work through your fears. On the other hand, if something calms your mind into a sense of serenity, then try to trust in that process, even if it makes no rational sense to you right now.

You can strengthen your intuition by becoming aware of the space between your eyebrows. Closing your eyes and touching this spot known as "the third eye," will help you to access more of what your third eye "sees."

Meditation, deep breathing, and a willingness to explore the unknown also help you become more in touch with your own inner wisdom and guidance.

Once you practice following intuition, you will begin to notice ever-subtler "clues." Some people experience these as signs or synchronicity, while others cannot explain their feelings at all. Spiritually, something just "feels right" or "feels a little off."

Trust that *still small voice,* which quietly steers you into blessings and away from harm. By no accident has nearly every major religion developed a contemplative or mystic branch.

Whether you refer to your intuitive experiences as "ESP," "leading a charmed life," "answered prayer," "luck," or "good discernment," the fruits of turning inward bring with them a sense of something bigger, more mysterious, and more beautiful than ordinary life.

"Follow the Yellow Brick Road"

Information about brain injury travels slowly, even within the medical community. If you expect physicians and case managers to know all the answers, you will probably find yourself extremely disappointed. Even if other people do come through for you, waiting for those answers can cost you precious time.

This chapter focuses on actions you can take on your own.

11. Buy top quality electronics.

You are probably thinking *I don't know if I'll ever be able to work again, and this woman is telling me to spend money. Lots of it. Is she nuts?* No.

Actually, I speak from experience. Given that a majority of people with neurological problems either completely lose the ability to work on a computer or find the process extremely fatiguing, you may also benefit from this advice.

When I attempted graduate school after TBI, I bought the best monitor I thought I could afford: a Trinitron, with minimal flicker. I knew that the LCD panel of a laptop felt better on my eyes, but I did not think I could afford to buy one. The LCD flat screens for desktops had just hit the market, and I could not justify such a "luxury."

As a result, I dropped out of graduate school after only three weeks, in part due to headaches from my monitor. The slight flicker would sneak up on me, and if I spent too long on the computer, I saw flashing lights for several days.

My vision improved dramatically with visual therapy, but I still struggled with that monitor. Although I had much to say, I could not write for more than ½ to 1 hour a day. Even this assumed I was having "a good day" with plenty of sleep and not much other stimulation. I certainly could not count on my ability to do computer work on demand—not even in the controlled environment of my own home. These restrictions kept me disabled for years.

When I moved to Santa Fe in October 2002 my computer—mercifully—was destroyed in transit. I had always hated the set-up, and despite the expense, I felt glad to see it go. In an uncharacteristic splurge, I decided to buy a laptop. Unlike previous computer purchases dictated by my pocketbook, I chose this one for my health.

I cashed in a small IRA in order to pay for my laptop, which seemed scandalously expensive until I really thought about it. I had spent four and a half years unable to work and unable to write. Suddenly, it seemed like I had saved a few hundred dollars in order to lose a hundred thousand.

I added up all the writing or office work I could have done with a reliable monitor and realized I should have bought one years ago.

I have never once regretted my decision. I picked out the largest, best clarity screen I could find. It happened to be a Sony. For the top of the line screen, I got a top of the line laptop with far more memory than I ever thought I'd need. I may need all that hard drive after all: I now write four to nine hours every day.

In addition to allowing me to pursue my dream as a fulltime writer, the laptop lets me stay in better contact via email. It has opened a world of ancillary friendships that I never had the stamina to explore or maintain.

The laptop also provides mobility. If my home environment becomes too hot, too loud, or otherwise intolerable, then I can find another place to work. Sometimes it just feels nice to have people around or to sit outside in the sun. The flexibility of having a laptop accommodates my need for quiet, comfortable surroundings.

Another bonus: a built-in DVD player lets me watch movies and do yoga workouts without a television's annoying flicker.

Professor Stephen Hawking, the great physicist who has Lou Gehrig's disease, is mostly paralyzed and has lost control of his vocal cords. When walking became too difficult, he got a wheelchair; when he could no longer speak, someone designed a computerized "voice" for him.

Professor Hawking leads a more active and productive life than most "healthy" people. He travels around the world, giving lectures and writing books. He is one of the most respected physicists and great minds of our time. (You can read his personal story beginning in Appendix 3.)

Yet, without high quality electronics, Professor Hawking's genius would lie mute and immobile. What an incomprehensible tragedy and waste that would be! We live in a technological world: accept these gifts and journey onward!

12. Find ways to minimize stimulation.

The term "agnosia" refers to any sensory interpretation deficit. Following brain damage, many people lose the ability to distinguish between ambient noise and the primary conversation, or between the background and foreground of a visual scene.

Their formerly effortless system of filtration no longer works. What used to occur automatically now takes conscious effort. Consequently, people with TBI usually fatigue easily, especially in the presence of multiple stimulation.

If you suffer from any type of agnosia, you can compensate to some degree with external aids. Use earplugs in restaurants and crowds, so you can listen more easily to the people actually talking to you. Wear sunglasses if lights bother you. Avoid places with overhead fans, or do not face them. Wear comfortable clothing.

You can also buy a big, floppy hat to keep yourself from becoming overwhelmed. I used to wear a large hat whenever I wrote in coffee shops. The wide brim tuned out distractions, allowing me to devote full concentration to my laptop screen. I no longer need the hat, but wearing one helped me write over 100 pages of this book.

When selecting an apartment or house, you probably want to pay particular attention to the neighbors and any noises, smells or streetlights you might encounter. When calculating the cost of a location, consider how it will affect your health:

- If you cannot get a full night's sleep, then how will that play out in your ability to earn money the next day?
- If your neighbor's bass gives you a headache, then how does the cost of medication (sometimes up to $14 / pill) factor into your estimated rent or mortgage?
- If intense smells trigger reactions, then you may not want to rent or buy near a restaurant or garbage dump.
- If you suffer from Chronic Fatigue Syndrome or Fibromyalgia, you will particularly want to avoid places with an obvious mold problem.

Safety might become a larger concern than it was before your health turned south. Attacks cause trauma to anyone, but can you physically afford another blow to your brain? If you no longer drive, then the proximity of stores, restaurants, and public transportation will also become important.

Of course, aiming for total control of your environment will not allow you to live a normal life. Part of your recovery will include learning to tolerate other people's schedules and needs. You cannot prevent an occasional surprise, but you *can* maintain comfortable surroundings that help you deal with change.

13. Breathe slowly and fully.

Diaphragmatic breathing relaxes the entire body and brain. When you inhale, do not trap your breath in your chest. Instead, inhale all the way into your belly.

I've listed below some good exercises to get you started. You can practice these techniques at any time, set to relaxing music or in silence. You might even want to make your own guided meditation tapes by recording the instructions for yourself.

In moments of stress or pain:

- Concentrate on your breath filling the belly area.
- When you exhale, release all the air before your begin the next inhalation.
- Try to exhale for twice as long as your inhalation.
- Repeat until your breathing remains slow and calm on its own.

To clear anger or intense pain:

- Breathe in through your nose.
- Hold the breath for a few moments.
- Exhale through your teeth.
- Force all the negativity out with your breath.
- Inhale fresh, clean air through your nose.
- Repeat, releasing the anger or pain by exhaling through your teeth, easing with each cycle of your breath.

To clear anxiety and lower your heart rate:

- Lie flat on your back, arms at 45-degree angles, palms up.
- Slowly breathe in.
- Follow the breath through your nostrils and into the body.
- Feel the breath all the way into the belly.
- Sense your belly rising and falling with your breath.
- Let go.
- Let your body melt into the ground, feeling the Earth's support.
- Remember, you are not alone! Feel the support around you and let your worries evaporate.
- Remain in this position for at least one minute, or as long as you desire. Pay attention to your body. Then carry this feeling into your

day, remembering that you can access peace and relaxation whenever you need them simply by following your breath.

"Alternate nostril breathing."

Sit with a straight spine and relax your head forward until your neck feels just slightly stretched. Close your eyes.

- With your right hand, hold your ring finger over your left nostril and your thumb over your right nostril.
- Block off the left nostril and inhale slowly through the right.
- Block off both nostrils for just a moment to create a "space between your breaths."
- Then block just the right nostril and exhale slowly through the left.
- Now, inhale just through the left nostril.
- Block both nostrils again, and exhale through the right nostril.
- Repeat for several more cycles.
- When you finish, your mind will feel calm and clear.

Although this is an ancient technique, I first learned it from a Yogiraj Alan Finger CD called, "Life Enhancing Meditations." On this CD, he directs you through this and other meditations.

Use any of the above techniques to calm the mind and strengthen the love and natural connection between your body and your mind.

Breathing into pain with loving attention allows you to move faster and more easily through its grip. Relaxing your mind allows you to make informed choices rather than mere reactions to a momentary fear or pain.

14. Do the cross-crawl.

A number of physical exercises encourage communication between the right and left sides of your brain.

Cross-crawl:

- Get on your hands and knees.
- Move your right hand and your left knee forward at the same time.
- Repeat with the opposite sides.
- Move forward several times, using alternate hands and knees.
- Then, practice moving backwards.

When this becomes easy, you can practice on a hardwood floor or patterned rug, aiming for specific spots with hands and knees.

Cross-over Leg Kicks:

If you are relatively agile, you can also stand up and kick your legs like a Rockette, making sure to cross over the midline of the body. Crossing over helps to balance the left and right sides of your brain.

Less Mobile Options:

- If you find crawling uncomfortable or impossible, then you can take up knitting, which also coordinates right and left hemispheres.
- Alternatively, you can touch your right hand to your left knee and vice versa. Repeat 20-50 times per day, especially when brain function seems low. I have observed people in a scattered condition perform this exercise and immediately transform into lucid conversationalists.

Mental Exercise:

If you are in a public place or find it impractical to try any of the above exercises, you can simply *imagine* **your left and right brain having a conversation with each other:**

- Are they friends or enemies?
- Do they even recognize one another's existence?
- They share the duplex of your skull: perhaps it's time they become acquainted with each another.

- Do they have names?
- You can take this visualization as far as you desire, or you can just quickly acknowledge the importance of your *entire* brain.

In any case, when the "guy on the left" marries the "girl next door," you will experience better communication and understanding between the two hemispheres of your brain. This marriage of left and right creates and nurtures healing on all levels.

15. Practice yoga.

I once considered yoga too "woo-woo" to be taken seriously. Then I found myself unable to work out at a gym anymore. As muscle tone disintegrated, I searched for ways to get back in shape. Credited by Madonna for her arms and abs, yoga seemed gentle enough for my injured neck and brain.

I never expected the mental and physical relief. Unable to afford treatment for my neck, I was surprised and pleased when yoga gradually eliminated chronic spasms. The meditative aspect also eased my oversensitivity and migraines.

Yoga emphasizes self-acceptance, making it an ideal therapy for someone recovering from TBI or long-term illness. The new confidence in my ability to hold poses helped repair doubts about my body's ability to function properly again. (For additional comments about healing through yoga, please see the interviews with Robin Cohn and Sarah Kramer in Appendix 3.)

Yoga Terms defined:

Yoga: From the Sanskrit "yug," meaning "union" or "to yoke," yoga is a system of positions, breath and concentration that works to unite body, mind and spirit. When practiced regularly, yoga encourages relaxation, strength and flexibility.

Asanas: The positions or "yoga poses." These increase flexibility, develop balance, massage internal organs, and encourage your glands to secrete hormones, thereby helping to heal and detoxify your body.

Ashtanga yoga: Also known as "Power Yoga," ashtanga links the various asanas in a rapid flow sequence, providing an aerobic workout that increases strength and flexibility. Ashtanga may be difficult to follow if you do not already know the basic poses. Once you learn the asanas, performing these sequences can help you process life's other sequential requirements.

Bikram yoga: Developed by Bikram Choudhury, Bikram yoga demands a vigorous sequence of 26 poses performed in a very hot room. Classes move quickly and encourage the body to sweat profusely, removing toxins through the pores.

Although many students rave about the results of Bikram, in my opinion, this form of yoga is too intense for people with TBI. The extreme nature of both the classroom environment and the flow sequence might cause fatigue and disrupt your sensitive system. Not to mention the smell!

Hatha yoga: The form of yoga most commonly practiced in the West. In hatha yoga, the practitioner focuses on the breath, while holding various *asanas* for extended periods of time. You can learn hatha yoga poses from a book, if the idea of classes intimidates you.

Iyengar yoga: The path of yoga developed by B.K.S. Iyengar. Emphasizing precise body alignment using props like blocks and straps, Iyengar yoga helps people with injuries or inflexibility gain maximum benefit from the *asanas*.

Iyengar classes usually move slowly, with the instructor adjusting each student's posture and alignment. For this reason, an Iyengar yoga class offers a safe haven for someone recovering from an injury or illness.

Kundalini yoga: While all yoga aims to raise and embrace humanity's dormant "kundalini" energy, kundalini yoga (KY) claims to activate this energy 16 times faster than hatha yoga. Developed in India and Tibet over 50,000 years ago, KY gave birth to all other forms of yoga.

As brought to the West in 1969 by Yogi Bhajan, KY strongly emphasizes the spiritual aspects of yoga and encourages people to live "healthy, happy, holy" lives. Usually done with the eyes closed, KY can rapidly improve concentration and provide a sense of lightness and well-being.

I *love* kundalini yoga! However, it can become both physically and spiritually intense. Explore this form of yoga cautiously, especially if you have a neck injury or do not feel grounded on your own spiritual path.

You probably want to practice kundalini yoga with an instructor, rather than experimenting on your own; however, *www.kundalini.org* does offer free online classes. Of the DVD's available, I most recommend *Kundalini Yoga with Gurumukh*. She is truly a delight to the soul, and she leads one heck of a workout!

Mudras: Ritualized positions of the hands, frequently used in meditation. Different mudras activate different parts of the nervous system, producing a variety of physical, mental, emotional and spiritual effects.

Sivananda yoga: Deriving its roots from hatha yoga, Sivananda yoga explores five points in every class: relaxation, exercise, breathing, diet, and positive thinking. Newcomers to yoga often find Sivananda classes particularly supportive and instructional.

Vinyasa: The linking of breath and movement, *vinyasa* urges practitioners to pay attention to their breathing. Learning to move with our breath automatically attunes us to a more natural rhythm of life. Each action requires a breath, and each breath produces an action. When practiced properly, vinyasa teaches the importance of patience and persistence, and strengthens our faith that today's small steps make essential contributions to a larger process.

Vinyasa also helps retrain your left-brain's sequential thought.

Recommended video and DVD selections:

If you cannot find or afford a yoga instructor near you (or if you fear being photographed by your insurance company's private detective), there are many ways you can enjoy yoga at home. *Yoga Journal* offers a wide selection of relaxing and invigorating yoga videos. I particularly recommend the following 20-minute *Yoga Journal* classes:

- *Yoga for Stress Relief*
- *Lower Body Yoga for Beginners*
- *Power Yoga for Beginners for Stamina*

Sarah Bates, an Occupational Therapist, Fibromyalgia sufferer, and yoga instructor, has designed a yoga DVD specifically to meet the needs of disabled viewers. Sarah's DVD contains exercises you can perform in bed or in a chair, along with more vigorous workouts as viewers improve their technique and stamina. You can find out more about Sarah and "accessible yoga" on her website: *www.downwarddogproductions.net.*

Please note that my *process* of learning yoga was probably as important as the exercise itself. Something like Tai Chi or Qigong might have had an equally strong impact on my growing awareness of body, breath and energy. If you feel drawn to a particular form of meditative exercise, then trust your intuition, talk to your physician and enjoy.

16. Search for patterns.

In time, behavior, dreams, symptoms, and life situations: patterns can make you aware of important information. Tracking your emotional and physical states may show correlations between a behavior and certain symptoms. Paying attention to synchronicity, or "meaningful coincidences," helps clue you in to life's little nudges in a particular direction.

The enforced lack of busyness after my injury enabled me to notice repetitions of seemingly random people, places, or thoughts. I found that three unusual pointers in one direction would grab my attention. If I ignored the synchronicity, then the coincidences became more striking.

For example, I felt an urge to move to Seattle but could not explain why. When I dismissed the feeling, a neighbor moved in *from* Seattle; then my brother's roommate vacationed in Seattle; I "randomly" tuned into a radio program broadcast from Seattle; the first TV program I turned on in months happened to be a documentary on Mt. Rainier.

Over time, I learned to "listen" more closely. I eventually moved to Seattle, where I found an unusually effective combination of treatment providers. I also met the love of my life there. Coincidentally, given this *Wizard of Oz* theme, Seattleites often refer to their town as "The Emerald City."

Specifics:

- Keep track of recurrent symptoms and strenuous activities on a calendar.

  (When I suspected that reading and driving aggravated my migraines, I recorded the number of miles I drove or the number of minutes I read on any given day. After a few weeks, it became clear that I could not drive more than 30 miles in a week without a full-blown headache. For over a year, I could not read more than 5 minutes a day or 25 minutes in a week. Obviously, I had to keep rather abbreviated records, but the information allowed me to track my symptoms and progress.)

- You can also monitor food, medication, and intake of caffeine, looking for possible side effects.
- Whenever you experience unusual synchronicities, record them, along with the date and anything you can remember of surrounding circumstances. Keeping a record will help you analyze patterns. Perhaps as important, the written documentation serves as "proof" if you ever doubt your memory of events.

"If I Only Had a Brain"

The lack of public knowledge about TBI, combined with the need to avoid over-stimulation can turn recovery into a lonely and monotonous experience.

This chapter offers ideas to improve brain function and combat boredom. It also emphasizes that you are not alone on your journey.

Just as post-concussive Dorothy finds companionship, you too can find inspiration and a support community.

17. Cultivate relationships with animals.

Dorothy's Toto offers constant companionship. He also recognizes the true nature of people like Miss Gulch, the Cowardly Lion, and the Wizard. Many pets exhibit uncanny sensitivity to human suffering. If you are lucky enough to have a pet, I encourage you to accept its nurturing. You can also connect with animals in the wild.

The effects of my TBI forced me to spend weeks recuperating at my parents' house. The nausea, confusion, and perpetual migraine headaches left me unable to do much but sleep for 16 hours a day, listen to Chopin, and eat whatever food my queasy stomach could handle.

I passed my first few weeks there in an alternately excruciating and euphoric haze, but by mid-June, I developed an afternoon routine. With Chopin lulling my brainwaves, I boiled water and heated two scones in the toaster oven. Struggling to walk with a cup of tea in one hand and the scones in the other, I would sink into the back porch chaise—exhausted once again.

I was often too tired to feel my boredom, but occasionally it surfaced in anguishing waves of isolation. My parents worked during the day, so when I awoke at 1p.m. I had no companionship. Nor could I focus my attention enough to read or meditate. In fact, almost any stimulation sent me reeling into vertigo, but the lack of conversation or distraction felt unbearably lonely.

Somewhere in the course of those back porch afternoons, I noticed what looked like an owl sitting on a branch at the end of my parents' property. Day after day, it returned.

When the thought finally occurred to me that owls do not usually show themselves in daylight, I considered I might be hallucinating. With intermittently double vision and all those painkillers, it certainly seemed possible.

Still, I came to enjoy my afternoons with this owl, who so reliably settled on the same branch—always within a few minutes of my thud into the chaise. He was the perfect companion: quiet, knowing, keen of sight.

I never spoke to him, nor he to me, yet we developed an understanding between us. I could feel his presence, even with my eyes closed. Although the crows harassed him mercilessly, he sat with me for as long as I remained outside.

One Saturday, my mother decided to lounge on the back porch as well. I stretched out and began to anticipate the owl's company. My mom suddenly hissed in excitement: "Laura, that looks like an *owl*! Back there, in the trees. I have to go get my binoculars." She ran into the house and came out with them around her neck: "Oh my Go—It *is*. A great horned owl! But what's it doing outside at 3:00 in June?"

As she gazed through her binoculars, I nonchalantly explained to her, "He's my friend. He sits with me every day when I come out here."

"What!?" My mom was now surprised and envious. A longtime collector of owls, she had joined the Audubon Society in hopes of seeing more of them in the wild. "Laura, why didn't you tell me?"

I answered her truthfully, "Because I wasn't sure if he was real."

Eventually, I recovered enough to return to my own apartment, and my mother never saw the owl again. Curiously, she did *hear* the owl on certain nights, but only when I happened to be visiting their home again. Over the years, it has become a joke between us that when I arrive, "my" owl welcomes me.

On a visit home, I had a strange dream of two dark, catlike figures that were not cats. They danced an elaborate S-pattern and then melted into one another. I had no idea what the dream might symbolize, and yet it seemed important—like in dreaming it, I had participated in a ritual of wholeness.

At breakfast, I described the dream to my mom, and she did not know what to make of it either. She went upstairs to fold laundry and abruptly yelled for me to come up there. She stood looking outside the window at some disturbances on the previous night's snowfall. "Laura, I think we need to go outside and check this out."

We bundled up and trudged through the snow to the markings she had noticed from above. Two sets of tracks in S-like patterns appeared as if out of nowhere. Judging by the direction of the toes, two large birds had dropped from the sky and undulated towards one another on the ground. After coming together, they once again took flight.

Of course, I cannot say with certainty that it was my old companion, but great horned owls do begin their courtship in late January. I like to think our bond remains. A true friendship: no matter how long the separation, we share key moments in our lives.

Since my injury, I have noticed unusual responses from many animals. When in the process of making an important decision, I frequently see one or three bald eagles. Dogs sit with just a look from me; normally skittish cats climb into my lap. The animals seem to understand what humans miss. This enhanced relationship with animals has become one of the greatest blessings of my TBI experience.

18. *Initiate new friendships.*

Although now may not seem like the time to seek out new friends, this is exactly what you should be doing. I'm not suggesting you become a social butterfly—only that you do not resist people's attempts to befriend you in your current situation. **I urge you to make new friends for a variety of reasons:**

- You can use all the support you can get.
- Your old friends might have difficulty accepting the changes in your life.
- Your old friends might feel so sorry for you that they instigate depression.
- New friends will accept you as you are, instead of comparing you to your "old self."

I remember how embarrassed I felt when I realized I could no longer participate in my friends' intellectual discussions. A few friends remained supportive throughout my entire recovery, but most lost patience with my high-maintenance requirements for socializing.

I always needed a ride, and if a migraine developed, then I needed to be taken home immediately. I could not watch movies in a theater. Even on a VCR, I could only view films in a fully lighted room.

Sometimes in the middle of a conversation, my tolerance for noise evaporated, and I demanded my friends' sudden and absolute silence until I recalibrated. Any flicker or moving visual background made me so nauseous and dizzy that I avoided nearly every store or restaurant—except on a *very* "good day."

The friends I kept tended to live several hours away, so they rarely saw me at my worst. I rested several days before they visited in order to make it through an afternoon without my nap.

Although some friendships ended because of my friends' discomfort, pity, or impatience, most fizzled because we simply grew apart. So much of my pre-injury life had revolved around literature, graduate programs and traveling for work, that when I suddenly became a nonintellectual homebody who could not read, we had little left in common.

My TBI served as an indicator of what sort of friendship I had with each person. If the friendship had arisen from convenience rather than through a meeting of the souls, then it did not survive the change. If the connection ran deeper than shared activities, the friendship evolved.

After I overcame my initial reluctance to meet new people, I discovered that they generally accepted and admired me. I had wrongly assumed that anyone who had not already loved me could not possibly want me as a friend. Why would they want to connect with someone so restricted?

Due to my own insecurities about the injury, I always told people about my TBI within a few minutes of conversation.

Before they invested in me, I wanted them to know that they could walk away. Few did. I found instead that people wanted to learn what kept me going.

I became their source of inspiration, and they became companions on my journey. We developed symbiotic relationships, in which they drove me places or paid for meals, while I told stories and provided spiritual insights to their problems.

I never would have expected it, but two years post-injury, I had developed closer and deeper friendships than I had ever had pre-injury. And lots more of them.

Amidst all the pain, fatigue and limitations of TBI, time stood like an open plain. Whereas before the accident, I needed to squeeze friendships in between business trips or term papers, afterwards, I could devote myself entirely to two things: getting well and listening to my friends.

So long as the two did not conflict, the connections flourished. Only when someone demanded more than I could give—in other words did not accept me with my vulnerabilities—did I pull away. For the most part, my post-injury friends brought laughter, joy and companionship to what would otherwise have been a terribly lonely road.

Even if you choose not to initiate friendships right now, know that you are not alone:

- The Scarecrow—no brain
- Dorothy Gale—concussion
- Jake Barnes in Hemingway's *The Sun Also Rises*—concussion
- Louisa Musgrove in Jane Austen's *Persuasion*—head trauma
- Star hockey player client in *Jerry Maguire*—4 concussions
- James Brady (President Reagan's Press Secretary)—TBI
- Dick Button (figure skating legend)—TBI
- Bob Dole (U.S. Senator)—TBI
- Goldie Hawn (actress)—TBI
- Chevy Chase (actor)—electrocuted
- Laura Hillenbrand (*Seabiscuit* author)—CFS
- Sarah Kramer (author of 3 best-selling cookbooks)—CFS
- Fyodor Dostoyevski (Russian novelist)—epilepsy
- Christopher Reeve (a.k.a. Superman)—spinal cord injury
- Stephen Hawking (physicist)—Lou Gehrig's Disease (ALS)
- Patricia Neal—stroke

- H.G. Wells (author)—epilepsy
- Harriet Tubman (abolitionist)—TBI
- Alexander the Great (Roman Emperor)—epilepsy
- Julius Caesar (Roman Emperor)—epilepsy
- Eric Lindross (hockey player)—multiple concussions
- Steve Young (NFL football player)—concussions
- Troy Aikman (NFL football player)—concussions
- 5.7 million Americans, plus nearly 2 million each year—TBI
- 4.7 million Americans, plus nearly 700,000 each year—recovering from stroke
- 7-10 million Americans suffering from CFS, Fibromyalgia or Multiple Chemical Sensitivities

19. Practice Mindfulness.

Sometimes a loss in IQ points actually becomes a bonus. We live in a world of multi-tasking, but brain injury usually puts a stop to that. Take advantage of the chance to focus your attention on a single task-at-hand.

For months, I could do no housework except water my plants. The necessity of reminding myself of each step in the process forced me to notice those steps. I watched the water fill the can, listening to its sound. I observed the leaves as moisture dribbled down their shiny surface. I paid attention to the soil. Because watering plants required every bit of my concentration, I learned to appreciate them more.

Instead of frustrating yourself with too much stimulation, try to accomplish one thing at a time. You will find more pleasure in the task and probably perform it better anyway.

If you are interested in deepening your Awareness, a wide variety of resources is available on the internet, in bookstores and sometimes at your local library:

- John Kabat-Zinn is probably the best-known teacher and researcher of mindfulness used to relieve chronic pain. Two of his video tapes provide a good introduction and guidance: *Mindfulness and Meditation (Stress Reduction)* and *Inner Awakenings-Guided Imagery to Quiet the Mind, Strengthen the Body and Soothe the Soul.*
- I also recommend Deepak Chopra's meditation CD called "The Soul of Healing," which helps you embrace the potential for conscious healing in every cell of your body.
- Sally Kempton's book *The Heart of Meditation* provides a comprehensive collection of stories and instruction to deepen your practice and Awareness.

20. *Listen to classical music.*

Ever hear of the "Mozart Effect?" Don Campbell, a musician, teacher and author of nine books, including the 1997 best-seller *The Mozart Effect,* has dedicated his life to revealing how music influences the mind and body. Numerous studies indicate that listening to classical music helps neurological development and reduces stress.

For more information, check out Don Campbell's website, *www. mozarteffect.com.*

I personally found that Chopin's *Nocturnes* offered a perfect combination of relaxation and distraction from pounding headaches. The melodies were complex enough to occupy my mind, but not so intricate to overwhelm me. I spent days listening to the same Chopin CD. The music eventually became so familiar that I could "hear" it in stressful situations and immediately calm down.

Experiment with artists that particularly touch your soul. You will know the selection works for you when it lifts you out of your pain and into momentary joy.

21. *Listen to books and lectures on tape.*

> "That is part of the beauty of all literature. You discover that your longings are universal longings, that you're not lonely and isolated from anyone. You belong."
>
> F. Scott Fitzgerald

> "Literature is my Utopia. Here I am not disenfranchised. No barrier of the senses shuts me out from the sweet, gracious discourse of my book friends. They talk to me without embarrassment or awkwardness."
>
> Helen Keller

Your local library may carry a large selection of audio titles ranging from poetry to recent best-sellers. For a "quick read," you can choose from many abridged editions, but good libraries usually carry full-length cassette series, too. If you cannot find the books you want at your local library, you can contact any of several organizations:

- Recording for the Blind and Dyslexic: 866-RFBD-585 or *www.rfbd.org*
- National Library Service for the Blind & Physically Handicapped: 202-707-0744
- Books on Tape: 800-521-7925 or *www.booksontape.com*
- Recorded Books, Inc.: 800-638-1304 or *www.recordedbooks.com*

Many local libraries also carry classes on tape. I highly recommend The Teaching Company's *Super Star Teachers Series.* If you missed college, want to remind yourself of information you used to know, or just want to learn something new, this series covers everything from Ancient Greek Mythology to Beethoven to The New Physics.

Keeping your mind active can stave off depression. You can encourage your brain to heal by teaching it new information and patterns. Plus, you'll be making good use of your downtime. Who knows? Maybe you will discover a new interest or vocation.

- The Teaching Company: 1-800-TEACH12 or *www.teach12.com*

Crabby Apple Trees

Sometimes reputedly healthy and beneficial things attack us when we least expect. The trees revolt when Dorothy and the Scarecrow try to pick their apples, and occasionally our "solutions" do more harm than good.

Pay attention to your response, not your expectation. Brain injury disrupts the natural function of your hormones and sensitivity filters, causing you to react to some medications, foods and therapies in ways opposite from their intended effect. Just because something looks good for you, does not mean it will necessarily agree with you. On the other hand, you may reap great benefits from some so called "unhealthy" dietary habits.

This chapter encourages you to observe and to evaluate what you put into your body. When in doubt, trust your experience.

22. *Check any medications for side effects.*

My first post-concussion headache was more intense than a migraine and lasted for 16 months. Unable to eliminate my pain, doctors tried to lessen it with a variety of migraine drugs. A behavioral optometrist later informed me that near double vision could explain the majority of my headaches. The listed side effects of my migraine drugs included "dizziness" and "visual disturbances." The drugs the doctors had prescribed to treat my symptom had actually *aggravated* its root cause.

Don't expect your doctor or pharmacist to discover all contraindications of your medication. Because brain injury symptoms vary so much among individuals, professionals may not have much experience with your particular issues. Moreover, they may not often work with people as sensitive as most TBI patients tend to be.

- One of the best resources is *The Merck Manual—Second Home Edition*, available in most bookstores and through online vendors.
- *The Merck Manual* provides comprehensive information on drug-drug, drug-food, drug-disease and dietary supplement-drug interactions.
- Your physician or naturopath probably owns *The Merck Manual*, so you may be able to consult it in their office, or at least ask them to consult it on your behalf.
- The Merck Manuals Online Medical Library also lists information on common drug-supplement interactions: *http://www.merck.com/mmhe/sec02/ch019/ch019a.html*. (Scroll down for the chart.)

As you can see, the information is available, just not always utilized.

23. Buy "Organic."

Some people develop extreme sensitivity after TBI. Pesticides, animal hormones and chemical preservatives can aggravate an already overloaded system. If you feel continually fatigued and overwhelmed, eliminating common toxins will help your recovery process. Once your system begins to relax, you can spend more energy on healing.

If your grocery store does not offer much organic produce, you can wash your fruits and vegetables with food-grade soap to ensure removal of all pesticides and wax. Some stores sell "veggie washes" and "veggie brushes" for this purpose or you can order products online. If you eat a great deal of frozen or packaged food, buy fresh produce and see if you feel any better.

People who eat meat, eggs and dairy, will probably notice the greatest changes when switching from ordinary products to organic versions. Traditionally raised chickens, pigs and cows ingest huge quantities of pesticides, antibiotics and hormones in farmers' efforts to promote fast growth and maximum productivity. These substances, particularly the hormones and pesticides, can wreak havoc on an already struggling endocrine system.

Before you rule out organic foods as way out of your budget, consider that organic fruits and vegetables contain denser quantities of nutrients than foods grown through traditional methods. Plus, they just taste better!

If nutritional content and taste do not convince you to buy organic, then perhaps the following information will: organic foods are *not* genetically modified organisms (GMO). What's a GMO? It means that a scientist created your "food" in a biotechnology laboratory, splicing genes from various organisms and combining them to make something entirely new and non-natural, but which masquerades as the real deal.

Sound like *Frankenstein*? More like those cannibals in Joseph Conrad's *Heart of Darkness*: one type of genetically engineered rice contains three human genes!

As creepy and sci-fi as it sounds, if you're not buying organic, then *most* of the food you ingest has been genetically altered to make it more marketable or profitable. This is potentially serious stuff! Types of genetically engineered (GE) corn, for example, are considered legal pesticides.

Yes, you read that correctly: *the GMO corn itself is a pesticide*. Some of the most questionable GE foods have been relegated to animal feed, but if you eat meat fed GE food, then you're still eating the consequences of unnatural foods—just higher up the food chain.

In a June 3, 1994 article, Joseph E. Cummins Professor Emeritus (Genetics) Dept. of Plant Sciences University of Western Ontario explained:

"The majority of crop plant constructions for herbicide or disease resistance employ a Promoter from cauliflower mosaic virus (CaMV). Regardless of the gene transferred, all transfers require a promoter, which is like a motor driving production of the genes' message. Without a promoter, the gene is inactive, but replicated, CaMV is used because it is a powerful motor which drives replication of the retrovirus and is active in both angiosperms and gymnosperms. The CaMV pararetrovirus replication cycle involves production vegetative virus containing RNA which is reverse transcribed to make DNA similar to HIV, Human Leukemia Virus and Human hepatitis B. (Bonneville et al. RNA Genetics Vo.11, Retroviruses, Viroids and RNA Recombination pp. 23-42, 1988). CaMV is closely related to hepatitis B and is closely related to HIV (Doolittle et al. Quart.Rev.Biol. 64,2, 1989; Xiong and Eickbush, EMBO Joumal 9, 3353, 1990)." http://www.psrast.org/jccamv.htm

In other words, the GE process often uses genetics from some of the worst diseases we know. Many consumers unknowingly eat close genetic variants of these diseases everyday. For example, GMO soya forms one of the highest percentages of processed foods, with no requirements to label the soy as GMO. It then becomes filler in animal feed, enchilada sauce, candy bars, TV dinners, or any number of packaged foods.

This means that unless you're eating something labeled "non-GMO" or "organic," then it more than likely contains a promoter related to HIV, Human Leukemia Virus, and Hepatitis B. Companies research and develop foods so quickly that no one really knows the long-term effects of our unnatural food chain.

It's enough to make one wonder, though.

24. *"Let your food be your medicine."*

Hippocrates, the founder of Western Medicine, famously said, "Let your food be your medicine and your medicine be your food." Increasing your intake of fresh, uncooked fruits and vegetables will dramatically increase your body's ability to repair itself.

Moreover, eating an apple requires almost no preparation, saving you the energy needed to cook all your meals. Try throwing some fruit into a blender for two minutes, creating a luscious smoothie for breakfast or a snack. Some grocery stores sell bags of organic baby carrots that you can munch on instead of chips. Organic celery sticks offer another great, highly mineralized snack option.

Eating fresher foods will increase your energy in several ways:

- By saving energy normally used for lengthy food preparation
- By giving your body more nutrients
- By eliminating common toxins
- By eliminating more difficult to digest foods

If you have a health food store or juice bar near you, you might also want to treat yourself to fresh juices—especially wheat grass juice—several times per week. Fresh juices can be expensive, but you will appreciate the jolt of energy and immediate sense of well-being they create. Wheat grass juice contains such concentrated amounts of vitamins and minerals that you would need four pounds of organic vegetables to obtain equivalent nutrition to just two ounces of this little green liquid!

Fish are called "brain food," because they contain Omega-3 Essential Fatty Acids (EFA's). This kind of fat supports brain function, helps concentration, and may even lessen symptoms of depression. Some research indicates that Omega-3 EFA's also act as natural anti-inflammatories and help to manage pain.

Although scientists have recommended fish for many years, recent studies show large concentrations of toxic chemicals in fish. Unfortunately, side effects of mercury toxicity include neurological problems, perhaps reinforcing the very symptoms you hope to cure. You might want to eat fish in moderation, or consult your doctor.

If you are vegetarian, allergic to fish, or concerned about mercury poisoning, experiment with oils from flax seeds or walnuts: both contain Omega-3's. Soaking nuts and seeds for several hours or grinding them dry makes them easier to digest.

You can benefit even more by combining Omega-3's with the Omega-6 EFA's contained in Evening Primrose or Borage Oils. **Hemp seed oil contains a naturally perfect blend of Omega-3's and Omega-6's.** Crystal Manna™ and E3Live™ are two supplements that also contain EFA's, along with amino acids, minerals and rare trace nutrients. Made of special algae from the waters of Klamath Lake, Oregon, these potent superfoods are an acquired taste with the potential to supercharge your brain.

I have never found any official research on the subject, but it has been my own experience and that of clients recovering from trauma, that increased protein intake helps brain function. Although mostly vegetarian pre-injury, I eagerly devoured four steaks the first week after I hit my head. The meat helped ground me when nausea and vertigo sent me reeling.

Experiment with what works for you, recognizing that your preferences may change as you heal.

Health food and fitness stores offer a variety of protein supplements, including hemp seed, rice, and "green food." I do not use soy or whey (dairy) protein supplements. Most whey protein is not organic, so it also includes pesticides, antibiotics and hormones fed to the cow, and dairy can cause major allergy symptoms. Not everyone tolerates soy: some people experience gas, acne, hormonal irregularity, foggy thinking, and slow metabolism when they ingest too much soy.

For these reasons, I emphasize hemp seeds, hemp protein powder, NutriBiotic™ brand rice protein, or "superfoods" like spirulina, maca, raw cacao, and wheat grass juice. If you prefer vegetarian whole foods rather than supplements or meat, then make sure you eat a wide variety of legumes/sprouts, vegetables, whole grains and dark leafy greens to ensure you meet all your nutritional needs.

On the opposite side of the spectrum, you might want to see how you feel when consuming primarily raw fruits, vegetables, nuts and seeds—a relatively *low* protein diet. Digestion of cooked foods, particularly cooked flesh and dairy, uses vast reserves of energy and creates toxic byproducts.

A grilled chicken dinner can take as long as 100 hours to digest! Even then, the digestion will probably remain incomplete, because heat destroys enzymes that occur in food's natural (uncooked) state.

Each raw food carries its own specific enzymes for digestion. When we destroy these enzymes through cooking, our pancreas needs to work overtime, creating "digestive enzymes" to break down food. (Humans have the largest pancreas relative to body weight in the entire animal kingdom.)

The pancreas eventually grows fatigued, leaving foods inadequately digested when they reach the intestines. Food allergies, constipation, "fogginess," fatigue, heartburn and migraines can result.

The enzymes in raw foods remain intact, so that your body does not need to produce additional enzymes to digest your meal. (Soak nuts and seeds in water, to deactivate "enzyme inhibitors.") Despite offering only a few grams of protein per serving, leafy greens like kale, spinach, cabbage, and romaine lettuce contain some of the most easily and completely absorbed amino acids available.

Amino acids are the building blocks of protein and are necessary for every metabolic function. With shorter, easier transit times in the digestive tract, raw food allows your body to spend more energy on healing. (If you like or feel you need meat and cooked food at this time, digestive enzyme supplements with meals can take some of the burden off your digestive system, thereby freeing more energy for healing.)

If you would like to learn more about a raw food lifestyle, the internet offers some excellent resources. Key in "raw food" on Google or Yahoo! for thousands of results. Some good raw food websites are:

- *www.rawglow.com*
- *www.shazzie.com*
- *www.alissacohen.com*
- *www.rawfamily.com*

The creator of rawglow.com suffered from Chronic Fatigue Syndrome and found powerful relief from a raw diet.

Shazzie cured herself of depression and netted a fortune!

Alissa Cohen resolved her Fibromyalgia by switching to a 100% raw food diet. Her book, *Living on Live Food*, shares information on starting and maintaining a raw food diet. She also offers a two-DVD set of "un-cooking" demonstrations.

People with difficulty following a linear recipe might find the DVD's easier to follow. Before recovering, I know I learned much better through demonstrations than by reading. You can watch small sections at a time, so you don't get overwhelmed. Then, after each section, you can make some quick, simple and delicious food right away if you already own a blender. (You may need fancier equipment like a dehydrator for some of the later recipes.)

Another easy, inspirational and *larger print* un-cookbook is Sergei and Valya Boutenko's *Eating without Heating*. Their mother, Victoria Boutenko also offers *Green for Life*, a book about the easy healing power of green smoothies.

- Tip: wear earplugs when using a blender or food processor!

Can't be bothered by all that blending and chopping?

- Check out *www.oneluckyduck.com*, where you can purchase premade, organic, enzyme-rich treats to enhance your diet.

I did not discover the advantages of a high (80%-100%) raw diet until I had almost fully recovered from my TBI; however, the difference in mental clarity, elevated mood, and increased energy shocked me. I experimented with "cooked" and "raw" days:

- When I ate cooked food, I usually needed an afternoon nap, struggled with irritability and frustration, and felt my eyes working against each other.
- On "raw" days, I felt a sense of health and wellbeing, my vision seemed better, and I did not need a nap.

Experiment with how foods make you feel. For example, after gradually losing the ability to digest most plant proteins, I had nearly run out of foods to eliminate. In 2003 in desperation, I finally swore off dairy for two weeks to see if anything changed. Amazingly, most of my other food intolerances disappeared.

Keep experimenting: in this age of "wheat-free diets," I was surprised to recognize that I felt great eating lots of whole grain wheat, and yet *oats*—those sweepers of cholesterol so touted by the American Heart Association—always resulted in dark feelings of depression and anxiety the day after I consumed them.

Again, personal experience remains the key to deciding how diet affects your recovery.

That said, even if you believe you "cannot live" without diet soda and sugar-free treats, you might want to quit consuming anything with artificial sweeteners *immediately*:

- Aspartame, Equal®, NutraSweet®, and phenylalanine are all names for a ubiquitous neurotoxin known to cause dizziness, seizures, loss of vision, nausea, tinnitus (ringing in the ears), and even death.
- Aspartame releases methanol, which turns into formaldehyde—a known carcinogen.

- **According to some studies, many people diagnosed with Fibromyalgia, lupus or M.S. actually suffer Aspartame poisoning**. When they stop consuming diet sodas, their symptoms diminish or disappear. (For more information, please see: *http://www.sweetpoison.com/aspartame-articles.html.*)

If you suffer from any kind of neurological problem and add Aspartame to the mix, you risk further complications.

You can try safer, alternative sweeteners like:

- Agave nectar
- Stevia
- Yacon Syrup
- Xylitol

All sweeten foods without spikes in blood sugar or poisonous chemical reactions.

When you ingest large quantities of medication, pesticides, or artificial "foods" your liver works overtime, processing toxic residues.

Foods thought to support liver function include:

- Artichokes
- Arugula (also called Rocket)
- Beets
- Bok choy
- Broccoli
- Burdock root
- Cabbage
- Kale
- Lemon
- Sweet potatoes
- Spinach

Drink lots of purified water to encourage elimination through the kidneys and urinary tract as well.

You might also consider supplementing your diet with liquid chlorophyll. The taste is somewhat acquired, but chlorophyll helps to oxygenate the blood, including blood going to the brain. Certain medical tests can reveal if specific areas of your brain receive less oxygen than they should.

For example, a S.P.E.C.T. scan showed reduced oxygen in my right and left cerebellum. Had I known about liquid chlorophyll in May 1999, I would have taken it then to give my blood and brain an extra oxygen boost.

Chlorophyll can also help your body recover from anemia, which often contributes to ongoing fatigue. Not surprising given its superstar nutritional status, wheat grass juice contains about 70% chlorophyll.

25. *Learn to utilize natural remedies.*

If you decide to take herbal supplements, you must remember that they are natural and powerful *drugs*. Always list them when a doctor asks for current medications. If your physician does not use or believe in herbal remedies, then you must learn about contraindications on your own.

I found the following list of herbs and nutritional supplements useful at one time or another in my recovery. For your convenience, I include references to possible side effects, but these often vary among individuals. *Again, this is for informational purposes. I am not a doctor.*

- *Gotu Kola*: Used by yogis before meditation in order to balance the right and left hemispheres of the brain, gotu kola offers some obvious attraction for a TBI survivor. My herbalist introduced me to gotu kola about 15 months post-concussion, and I continued to take 450 mg / day for another 2 years.

Tired of spending so much money on supplements, I once tried to stop my gotu kola consumption. About a week later, my thyroid sped up so fast that I had to eat constantly just to maintain my weight. I could not sleep and felt strung out. As an experiment, I restarted my gotu kola supplements, and the symptoms ceased.

Psychological dependency? Perhaps. But the herb is non-toxic, and my vision and tolerance for stimulation seemed better when I used it. At about $5.00-$8.00 per month, I figured I could afford this one, eventually stopping it when I felt ready.

- *Baikal Skullcap*: Also known as Chinese skullcap, this herb is not the same as ordinary skullcap, which acts as a mild sedative. Baikal skullcap can help sleep, too, but it acts primarily to detoxify the liver. The Chinese believe a congested liver causes a person to fall asleep fine but awaken a few hours later with racing thoughts and difficulty falling back to sleep. Baikal skullcap can help treat this type of insomnia. It's a difficult to find herb, but some health food stores carry it, as do a number of online suppliers.
- *Gingko Biloba*: Most popularly touted as a memory enhancer, gingko is also a natural blood thinner. **Anyone on anti-coagulant medication** ***should not*** **take gingko, except under careful medical supervision.** I began taking ginkgo to help me adjust to Santa Fe's high altitude when I moved there from Seattle. I did notice increased energy and some sharpening of short-term memory.

Unfortunately, those around me also noticed a quickening of my temper. I felt constantly on edge, and people seemed to irritate me without provocation. When I stopped taking gingko, a persistent skin rash disappeared, along with my bad mood. I experienced a bit more forgetfulness but considered this a small issue compared to the nasty side effects. In other words, gingko (or that particular source of gingko) did not agree with me.

- *Ginger:* One of the most effective cures for nausea, ginger can be enjoyed in teas, food, or capsules. I took ginger every day for four years to quell the effects of constant vertigo. A mild anti-inflammatory, ginger can also take the edge off a headache or chronic pain. Combined with garlic and onion, ginger makes a powerful immunity booster.
- *Milk Thistle:* A gentle liver cleanser, milk thistle offers virtually no known side effects. Whenever my allergies or sensitivities increase to unbearable levels, I experience relief with 400 mg of milk thistle per day.
- *Burdock Root:* Another liver cleanser, burdock produces more intense results than milk thistle. I find it helpful to introduce cleansing herbs slowly, as "detoxification symptoms" can mimic early stages of TBI: vertigo, nausea, mental confusion, and fatigue. For this reason, you probably want to consult a nutritionist or herbalist before beginning any cleanse. Remember that you are trying to support your body, not provoke an additional stress response.
- *Licorice:* Considered an adrenal tonic, licorice is one of the most common ingredients in Chinese herbal formulas. Taken to ease symptoms of stress, licorice should nevertheless be **used cautiously or not at all by anyone suffering from ragweed allergies, hyperthyroidism, or high blood pressure.** Do not consume large quantities of licorice at one time, as its natural laxative action may keep you close to the bathroom for several days!
- *Skullcap:* Used as an occasional sleep aid, skullcap can offset the insomnia that so often follows TBI. Consult an herbalist or naturopath as to how long you can use this herb.
- *Valerian:* Known for its relaxing properties, valerian is another herbal sleep aid. For some reason, valerian does not always relax me. Sometimes it agitates and angers me, and my skin tends to break out afterwards. Again, your response is more important than what the herb purports to do.
- *Melatonin:* Not an herb, but a supplement touted as a sleep aid, melatonin is used by some people to combat jetlag. Taken an hour before bedtime, the compound affects serotonin levels in the brain, supposedly ensuring a good night's sleep. As with valerian, I did not

fare well with melatonin. I slept soundly for about 45 minutes, and then awoke. After four nights of lying in a wide-awake stupor, I opted for my natural insomnia.

- *Nutmeg*: Used as a spice or in capsule form, nutmeg induces relaxation. For a few weeks, I drank a rice milk / protein / nutmeg mixture about 20 minutes before retiring. It knocked me out for about four hours, at which point I would have to re-dose. The nutmeg left me slightly groggy the next day, but I felt well rested. I kept needing greater amounts to fall asleep, and eventually it stopped working at all. For occasional insomnia, though, this cupboard spice comes in handy. It is not recommended by herbalists for long-term use.

- *Kava Kava*: A sedative herb with narcotic effects. I personally would not recommend kava for people with TBI or balance issues. Again, I'm not a naturopath, but *whoa!* This is some potent stuff! When I accidentally took some as part of a Whole Foods smoothie, my vision doubled, and I could barely walk home. I felt as euphoric and disoriented as immediately after my concussion.

- *B-vitamins*: Many people in a high state of stress find relief from supplemental B-vitamins. In the proper dose, a good B-complex can support the neurological system. In too high a dose, the excess vitamins usually flow out in your urine. You may want to consult a nutritionist about the right amount of B-vitamins considering your diet and overall health. High levels of some individual B's, like niacin, can sometimes cause nerve pain and skin rashes.

- *Calcium and Magnesium*: These two minerals work together to flex and relax your muscles. We all know that too little calcium can result in osteoporosis, but fewer people know that too little magnesium causes tension. I know of several people who manage to avert migraines by dosing themselves with magnesium. Others find that a calcium/ magnesium supplement helps them fall asleep at night.

- *Potassium*: Hyperthyroidism, diet sodas, and some medications leach potassium out of the body, causing leg cramps or muscle weakness. Bananas provide an excellent source of potassium, as do potatoes. Believe it or not, those EmergenC™ packets that you add to water contain among the highest doses of potassium available in supplement form.

- *Zinc, copper and iron*: Some doctors have found that supplementing zinc in the diets of Fibromyalgia sufferers results in a dramatic reduction in all symptoms. Zinc, copper and iron work together and compete against one another within the body, so approach long-term zinc supplementation with caution. Blood tests can identify mineral imbalances, and then you can supplement if necessary.

For Merck's online chart listing common drug-supplement interactions, click the following link and scroll down:
http://www.merck.com/mmhe/sec02/ch019/ch019a.html.

26. Consider a Candida connection.

Candida albicans, also known as "yeast," co-exists with beneficial bacteria in our intestinal tract, on our skin, and quite literally all over our environment. If a doctor analyzed a stool sample from a "healthy" person, s/he would find *Candida.* So what's the problem here? The concentration of *Candida.*

Certain factors like antibiotic or steroid use, hormonal therapies (including birth control pills), excessive sugar or mold intake, and trauma or stress, disrupt the natural balance of intestinal flora (the bacteria that help us digest our food). When something kills the "good bacteria" that feed off yeast, then the yeast begin to take control.

Candida produces poisonous alcohols, formaldehyde and other toxins as byproducts of its metabolism and reproduction. As yeast takes over, these chemicals increase in the host's bloodstream.

Candida overgrowth has been linked to:

- Chronic Fatigue Syndrome
- The so-called "fibro-fog" of fibromyalgia
- Memory problems and depression
- Asthma
- Allergies (especially to smoke and mold)
- Weakened immune function
- Food allergies
- Hypersensitivity
- Multiple Chemical Sensitivity
- And a long list of other ills

Even if you have never experienced a vaginal yeast infection or thrush, *Candida* overgrowth can still play a role in your current medical complaints. Most yeast resides in the intestine and on the skin. The typically recognized yeast infection and thrush appear only when yeast has grown so numerous that it invades other parts of the body. In its fungal state, yeast can become systemic, invading vital organs, including the brain.

Chlorinated water, prescription drugs, fast-food diets, refined flour and sugar, and the antibiotics and hormones fed to livestock make yeast overgrowth a widespread problem in the U.S.; however, there is no quick and easy way to eradicate the little beasties.

The *Candida* defense system involves the release of over 80 known toxins, which then enter the host's bloodstream. Referred to as a "Herxheimer Reaction," this die-off period often brings on flu-like symptoms and a worsening of the original yeast overgrowth symptoms. Because things get so much worse before they get better, many people quit a *Candida* cleanse long before they have eliminated the problem.

The quicker one tries to eliminate yeast, the worse the die-off phase, so I recommend a gradual approach, particularly for people already suffering from some other form of trauma. Dietary changes and herbal preparations can help significantly, along with supplements of *acidophilus* and *bifidus*—although heat weakens their effectiveness.

I found Pau D'arco tea a mild tasting way to detoxify from yeast. Despite its slightly sweet, pleasant flavor, this tea must be consumed in moderation! After a few days of one cup per evening, I decided to up my intake to four cups per day. Big mistake! The next day, I felt like I had been run over by a truck, caught the worst flu of my life, and swallowed glue into my lungs—all at the same time. These symptoms lasted a week and a half, and then I suddenly felt clear-headed, energetic and "lighter." The cleansing process was disgusting and painful, but worth the effort. I also no longer suffer from seasonal or food allergies.

Many yeast experts recommend a cleanse and then a maintenance program—usually at least four months, followed by lifelong dietary caution. The internet offers myriad *Candida* resources, and a number of books focus exclusively on yeast's role in the decline of American health. *The Yeast Connection: A Medical Breakthrough* by Dr. William G. Crook, is a good place to start. Others find Donna Gates' *Body Ecology Diet (BED)* helpful, if a bit rigid: *www.thebodyecologydiet.com.*

27. *Indulge your senses—but not all at once.*

Essential oils like lavender and peppermint relax the nervous system with minimal side effects. Inhaled or rubbed directly on the temples and neck, these oils can ease muscle tension, thereby reducing headache pain. You can usually find essential oils at your local health food store. If not, try ordering them online.

If you have allergies to ragweed, use lavender with caution. Essential oils of eucalyptus, cedarwood and clary sage can also tame tension, so long as they do not aggravate your allergies.

Drinking a cup of chamomile tea with candlelight and soft music in the background might sound incredibly relaxing. Just make sure the flickering candle does not disorient you.

If you decide to take a bath, then you will want to keep the room well ventilated. Some TBI survivors experience difficulty regulating body temperature. If a bath leaves you so overheated that you grow faint, dizzy, or sick, it defeats the purpose.

Massages can also induce relaxation—or over-stimulation. Opt for shorter sessions until you know your body and nervous system can handle an hour or more of touch. If you crave physical contact, I do encourage you to receive massages from practitioners or friends. Just be aware that even nurturing can be overdone.

"If I Only Had a Heart"

Cognitive problems seem like a logical side effect of brain damage, but TBI affects the entire person, including our emotions. Maybe you injured the specific part of your brain responsible for emotions. Perhaps you feel overall frustration and disappointment. If these feelings persist long enough, then you will need to recover from an injury *and* depression. This chapter encourages you to nurture yourself and to reach out to those around you. Little gestures can effect huge improvements.

28. *Find a balance in intimate relationships.*

Like any other form of trauma, TBI puts a strain on the most important relationships in our lives. No definitive guidebook navigates all the twists and turns of love between uninjured parties. Nor could one volume address all of the additional factors brought into a relationship by TBI.

Neurological problems, which directly influence our emotions and sense of identity, pose unexpected and unique challenges. Since TBI affects—and relationships occur between—individuals, I can only offer observations from my own experience.

Most people, no matter how well they knew you pre-TBI, will not understand your injury—at least not right away. Particularly if you look nearly the same as you did before, people close to you will struggle with their former expectations. They may "forget" or underestimate your injury so much that they grow frustrated at your seeming unwillingness to cooperate.

In a romantic relationship, such misunderstandings can cause deep pain on both sides. The changes in your personality and capabilities seem like a betrayal, and your partner's breaking heart may attack yours in self-defense.

TBI makes occasional ill-treatment unbearable. With all the things you have already lost, how can you afford a relationship that tears you down? On the other hand, your physical injury does not erase emotional history with each person in your life.

With the peculiar vulnerabilities that follow TBI, you probably do not want to make any irrevocable decisions. You might try to articulate how your symptoms feel, or how differently you now think.

In my experience, though, the people who love you most often put up blocks against understanding what has happened to you. Not because they do not care: they actually *want* to support you but find your situation too painful to acknowledge. *(See my essay in Appendix 3 for more on this topic.)*

Recognizing their dilemma helps. Of course, it seems unfair that you should have to consider their feelings when *you* suffered the injury, but human nature operates under its own rules. What people cannot hear from you, they may be able to hear from someone else.

Ask those close to you to read personal accounts and scientific articles about the TBI experience. Hearing other people describe similar issues validates your own struggle. If you belong to a TBI support group, you might want to invite your partner or spouse to one of the meetings.

- A number of excellent TBI recovery books exist, some even more appropriate for spouses, partners and families than for the survivors themselves. *Where is the Mango Princess?* by C. E. Crimmons is one such book.

- You can also encourage your caregivers to read Appendix 2 of this book—a section written by caregivers in support of other caregivers.

I wrote this book to appeal to family, friends and treatment providers as well as survivors. Once people glimpse "real" life after brain injury, they usually repent of earlier frustrations. Moreover, they will often become your strongest allies.

As for new romantic relationships, I recommend you proceed very slowly in matters of the heart. If you do become involved with someone early on, it helps to allow room for change. Having someone fall in love with you in your injured state can do wonders for your damaged self-esteem, and love's endorphins help battle depression.

On the other hand, if someone loves you exactly as you are, and the injured "you" is nothing like the healthy you, the relationship may impede your healing.

It takes a delicate balancing act to start a relationship after TBI, because you do not know how much you will recover. Ultimately, you may need to decide where your commitment lies: in a particular relationship or in maximum recovery.

For example, I developed a friendship with a man several months after I hit my head. His company eased many painful hours, and I know that his attention kept depression at bay. He also located the first doctor who really helped in my recovery and convinced my dad that my health was more important than financial security.

With overwhelming gratitude, I might say that I loved this man in a romantic way, except that "I" did not exist when we knew each other. He fell in love with the person he thought I was, but this version of me was like something out of a sci-fi movie. She looked like me, but had a much lower IQ, deferred all decisions to God or to other people, could not read, painted daily, lived in a complex mythological puzzle, and could only see him in her apartment three times a week. She looked real, but she was more like a ghost or doppelganger.

Ironically, the man who had spent so many months encouraging my recovery did not like the results at all. When my mind began to clear with visual therapy, he hardly recognized me.

I considered my progress a return to "normal," whereas he found me suddenly "uppity" and "inquisitive." In many ways, he reacted to my healing as others had reacted to the injury. The changes seemed like a bad mood swing, and he kept waiting for me to shift back to my docile "self."

We parted ways: according to him because I "might not recover," according to me because I had already recovered too much. I have often thought the story of our friendship makes for a good *Twilight Zone*.

So what *does* work in a relationship after TBI?

- Patience
- A sense of humor
- Keen observation (to know when a fight is due to symptoms)
- Flexibility
- Deep, unalterable love.

It takes a special person to be with a survivor of TBI, and it takes a special TBI survivor to provide mutual support and understanding to an uninjured person. The lines between health necessity, personal preference and selfishness often blur, and it takes open communication from both sides to find a balance.

Some things, like sleep, may become non-negotiable. Anything that interfered with a good night's sleep used to result in my nagging headache and quick temper the following day. My mind would shut down, and I resented any demands upon my time or attention. I could not demonstrate my love very well in that condition.

On both sides, it helps to see beyond our egos. My husband, Stephen, and I work daily to see each other in our entirety. It would be tempting to use my TBI as an excuse for my complexity, but we are all complex human beings. This means that Stephen has also experienced traumas that inform his behavior and expectations. Just as he needs to recognize the impact of TBI on my life, I need to accept him, too.

Unconditional compassion provides the deepest healing imaginable, but it requires hard work, honesty and vulnerability. The rewards of this type of relationship speak for themselves. They are the essence of all great love stories: finding that person who loves you for yourself and in spite of yourself. The one who loves you for who you really are.

Speaking from experience, great love stories are still possible after TBI. With curiosity, an open heart and the courage to love deeply, you really can find and generate amazing love.

29. Laugh more.

> "Then let us laugh. It is the cheapest luxury man enjoys, and,
> as Charles Lamb says, 'is worth a hundred groans in any state of
> the market.' It stirs up the blood, expands the chest, electrifies
> the nerves, clears away the cobwebs from the brain, and gives the
> whole system a shock to which the voltaic-pile is as nothing. Nay,
> its delicious alchemy converts even tears into the quintessence of
> merriment, and makes wrinkles themselves expressive of youth
> and frolic."
>
> —William Matthews

The old saying, "Laughter is the best medicine" actually has some truth
to it. Why does laughter feel so good? Some studies suggest that laughter
releases endorphins, which are natural painkillers, but only a little evidence
supports this physiological explanation.

Robert Provine, professor of psychology and neuroscience at the
University of Maryland has spent ten years researching laugher. He
concludes that laughter initiates and fortifies our sense of connection to
other people: "'We know that social support plays a role in everything from
healthy aging to cardiovascular disease. So at least in that regard, good
humor equals good health.'"*

Has your sense of humor changed with brain damage? Mine did.
Initially, my funny bone seemed inverted. If someone told a joke, I would
ponder the punch line for days, sometimes never getting it. Occasionally,
people told a joke, and I did not even know to look for a punch line.

On the other hand, I burst into loud giggles when no one else found
anything amusing. I couldn't help myself. Something would seem absurd—
probably because of my perceptual problems—and it would tickle me to
no end. If I recalled the situation weeks later, my laughter rolled again. I
changed from a lover of subtle irony to a huge fan of slapstick comedies.
Jim Carrey replaced Jane Austen. Television shows I had not deigned to
watch pre-injury suddenly became a favorite pastime.

Apparently, my response to TBI was not unusual. In a 1999 study,
Neuroscientist Robert Provine found that brain injured subjects often
have trouble finding punch lines, preferring instead slapstick or absurd
conclusions.

Sometimes, I still feel embarrassed by my silly humor, but I smile and
laugh a lot. Instead of taking offense, people usually seem amused and join

---

*   (Source: discovermagazine.com/2003/apr/featlaugh.)

me in "the giggles." Remember the song, "I Love to Laugh," from *Mary Poppins*? "The more I laugh—ha ha ha ha, the more I fill with glee. And the more the glee—hee hee hee hee—the more I'm a merrier me!" Everybody in the room rises to the ceiling on a wave of uncontrollable guffaws.

If you find something funny, by all means, laugh. Even if people have no idea why you are laughing, they will generally comment on your "great attitude" in the face of adversity. With all its restrictions, neurological mayhem also offers liberation. What feels more freeing than unabashed and childlike laughter?

30. *Celebrate.*

Whenever you pass a milestone in your recovery, it helps to acknowledge your progress and reward yourself. These steps forward can include anything from learning to walk again, to remembering your phone number, or returning to work part-time. It may seem silly to celebrate something that used to come so naturally to you, but remember how hard you worked to reach this point again.

Congratulate yourself as you "graduate" each level of recovery. If you cross a marker that gives you particular pride, invite others to share your joy. You might even want to have a little party or a fancy meal. Just do something to commemorate your progress.

Important anniversaries also merit recognition. My car accident occurred three days before my twenty-fifth birthday, making May 19 *and* May 22 rather loaded dates for me. I always tried to plan a special event around that time so that I did not focus on how much time I had "wasted" recovering.

Even when you recognize your progress and the blessings of the journey, anniversaries pose challenges. The calendar instigates unfair comparisons and what-ifs. I find it helpful to remember that I would have gotten older anyway—that at 30, I would have slowed down a bit from 25, with or without the injury.

Celebrating anniversaries takes a pro-active stance against depression. Instead of wallowing in self-pity, look for ways to mark the occasion in a fun and memorable fashion. Instead of considering how many months or years you have waited for health, honor how far you have already come.

31. *Learn to live from your heart & let go.*

"Think as I think," said a man,
"Or you are abominably wicked,
You are a toad.
"And after I had thought of it,
I said: "I will, then, be a toad."
—Stephen Crane 1895

And why *not* be a toad? Or at least someone who doesn't need to think all the time. I have always loved this poem, because it turns the judgment on its head. Try to embrace your situation and yourself with a sense of humor and an open heart. It takes effort to determine proper etiquette and self-expression—especially when TBI so radically challenges our concept of identity.

If our world-view can shatter with a simple bump on the head, then how accurate can our rational assessments be? Instead of trying to weigh out all the factors, listen to your heart. Observing the world with curiosity enables you to engage the world as you find it, without a preconceived belief system. This process promotes healing.

Compassion and non-judgment tend to have a ripple effect that far exceeds your original intention. For a few moments each day, close your eyes and connect with the world. Imagine waves of love radiating from your heart. Feel those waves join all the other waves around you. Feel yourself become one with the earth's natural vibration. Smile. Feel yourself evaporating, melting. Remember how it feels to have an open heart.

"I feel great! I've been holding that up for years," says Tin Man when he involuntarily drops his axe. After so much rigidity, his lubricated joints feel free. Instead of reacting to his lack of control, Tin Man embraces the chance to let go. You can too. TBI is a control freak's nightmare. On top of all the physical surprises and restrictions, you probably face employment, insurance and legal issues—none of which you can command.

Whenever friends or clients experience attacks from all angles, I ask them, "What are the odds of everything going wrong at once?" "I know," they say, "It's crazy" or "terrible" or "not fair." "Yes," I say, "But what are the odds?" Eventually, people recognize that the situation is probably not an accident. If all factors seem to converge against you, then you probably do not suffer from bad luck.

More likely, the universe has given you a chance to trust in its support. Only when every door slams in your face and locks, can you experience a miraculous exit. Without your hands tied and mouth gagged, you would not recognize the benevolence that circumvents your power. You can fight in vain to manipulate these situations, or you can abandon yourself to a love *that surpasses understanding*. If you let go, you will feel a touch of the Divine.

Have trouble getting out of your head and into your heart?

- Try Sally Kempton's *Awakened Heart* meditation CD.
- The CD, "*Novus Magnificat*" by Constance Demby, offers a stunning (though sometimes acoustically intense) soundtrack that opens the heart and supports meditative "journeying."

"Courage"

Poor Lion, he's such a bully. And why? Because he is afraid and has no pain tolerance. The mere thought of "what might happen" either paralyzes him or triggers an attack, thereby preventing any progress.

TBI can be incredibly terrifying. In one instant, you can no longer rely upon your brain's reactions. The world seems too fast, too loud, too bright. You don't know how or when you will recover. You might not know if you will ever work—or walk—again. Your insurance company might have a private detective on you. You might lose your lawsuit. Your doctors won't give you a prognosis. How will you learn to live with all this pain? What if it never goes away?

This chapter addresses the kinds of questions you try not to ask yourself—the ones that fester beneath the surface. The following hints are "courage boosters" and suggest ways to handle chronic pain.

32. *Write a letter to your pain.*

What might your symptoms be trying to tell you? Think of a cliché that corresponds to the location of your pain, i.e. "What a pain in the neck;" "I'm spineless;" "I just can't stay on my feet." How does this sentence apply to the habits or patterns in your life? The more obvious the cliché, the more important the message. View your pain as a messenger, not an enemy.

Once you have contemplated possible meanings of your injury, write a "break up" letter to your pain or symptoms. Thank them for all they have done for you, and kindly tell them you must now move on. Remember, your pain and symptoms think you need them. Let them know what you have learned from the experience and that you can live without their "help." Tell them the ways, if any, that you will miss them when they leave.

Remain firm and compassionate in your decision, just as you would in leaving a destructive friendship or relationship in life. You may have a long history with your pain and symptoms, but you have outgrown this companionship. Writing the letter will invoke your freedom.

The idea of physical imbalances representing mental, emotional, or spiritual issues dates back to ancient Sanskrit times. Six main nerve clusters, known as *nadis,* run up the center of the body. These *nadis* correspond to *chakras*, literally "wheels" of spinning energy. A seventh chakra spins just above the head.

Various spiritual and alternative traditions, including Reiki and yoga, have developed a system of awareness and healing that associates imbalances in the chakras with common physical, mental, emotional, or spiritual issues.

Recent medical studies have begun to confirm the association of each chakra with a particular endocrine gland. Imbalances in endocrine glands can in turn, coincide with emotional instabilities strikingly similar to the emotions associated with each chakra.

- For a good overview of the chakra system, please see *www.kundaliniyoga.org.*
- *Anatomy of the Spirit* by Caroline Myss (pronounced "mace") acted as a catalyst for me to become more in touch with my body and its messages. Around the two-year mark of my recovery, I stumbled upon this bestseller—available in print, audiocassette and video tape. Myss explores how connections among the seven sacraments, the Kabbalah Tree of Life, and the Hindu chakras influence our physical body.
- Another excellent resource is Louise Hay's classic book, *Heal Your Body,* an alphabetical listing of body parts and ailments matched to non-physical causes and suggested affirmations.
- *Want the results without having to learn all the details?* Relax! You can balance your chakras without knowing what they mean. Yogiraj Alan Finger offers amazingly transformative guided meditations in his CD, *Life Enhancing Meditations.*

IF I ONLY HAD A BRAIN INJURY

33. *Relinquish your attachment to recovery.*

In order to heal, you need to have Dorothy's commitment to find her home: "I'd give anything to get out of Oz altogether." Dorothy's determination to come back home overwhelms any doubt, fear, or fatigue she experiences along the journey. She commits herself to an unknown adventure, because she knows what she wants: a chance to live in the real world again.

She does not know that she will receive her wish, though. She follows the Yellow Brick Road with hope, not certainty. Each of Dorothy's companions on the way to the Emerald City asks her some variation of, "But what if I make the journey with you and the Wizard refuses to give me what I want?" Dorothy herself faces the same dilemma.

To the Scarecrow, she replies, "I couldn't say, but even if he didn't, you'd be no worse off than you are now." When debating whether or not to follow the road to recovery—or even to finish this book—ask yourself, *if you make the journey and wind up somewhere unexpected, would you be any worse off than you are now?*

By the time the Tin Man asks Dorothy about the Wizard's likelihood of granting him a heart, she replies with more faith, "Oh, but he will. He must. We've come such a long way already." She knows that they will walk away with *something*.

When the Cowardly Lion expresses doubts and fears about his ability even to ask for courage, Dorothy assures him that his friends will intercede on his behalf. She grows stronger and more determined on the course of her journey.

You will, too. Dare to hope the Wizard grants your wish, but recognize the value of your journey in and of itself. As your commitment grows, you become a wiser, more compassionate and courageous person. Many people with seemingly perfect lives cannot say the same.

Pioneers like you continued in the face of adversity, not knowing *what* the future held. They believed in the importance of their trek. Without pioneers, we would have no progress. Without a pioneering spirit, you will miss amazing friendships, experiences, and even—perhaps—your chance to heal.

34. *Express your vulnerability.*

Admitting your fears to yourself and people you can trust will go a long way in helping you to overcome them. If you are afraid to articulate what you are afraid of, then start there. Ask yourself (or ask God if that makes you more comfortable) to bring to consciousness your worst possible fear. Don't worry about overcoming it at this point. Just find out what it is.

Write it down or tape record it. In detail. Describe every angle of horror you can imagine happening to you if your fear came true.

- Is it one main fear, or a mess of smaller ones?
- Do some of them make you laugh when you put words to them?
- Which ones seem likely to occur?
- Look at the absolute worst-case scenario you have constructed.
- Could you live with that?
- How can you avoid it?

If the situation's outcome remains out of your control, then brainstorm ways of dealing with the worst-case scenario if it happens. Have you ever survived or even thrived when a nightmare came true? What happened?

Some fears may not disappear just because you write them down. If you still feel anxiety, find someone you trust and talk to them about your feelings. Ask them to listen to you first, without initially offering anything but support. Showing your weaknesses and fears to the right person can empower you.

Humans spend so much energy trying to hide our imperfections that we lose the sense of community. We also forget that shared vulnerability reveals courage and often earns respect instead of scorn. Traumatic events break down traditional barriers because social customs tend to hamper quick decisions about survival.

Chronic health issues place people in extended "survival mode." The ones who recover are not afraid to accept help when they need it.

35. *Try something new.*

The more creative or exciting this "something" is the better. Each day people with chronic health problems face a list of tasks they can no longer perform. Try something you never had time to do before your injury or illness. You may surprise yourself.

Years before my brain injury, I used to paint with acrylics. I had hardly taken this hobby seriously, though: I had never even bought a canvas! Frustrated by my inability to write, I knew I needed a creative outlet. I bought the largest canvas I could find and set to work.

To my surprise and delight, the picture turned out well. It became the first in a series that a few people have asked to purchase. Since I had never painted on canvas pre-injury, I had nothing former for comparison. This achievement stood on its own and gave me confidence. It also encouraged me to open my mind to other ways of earning a living.

When it seemed that I would never recover enough to work a traditional job, I tried to find something else I could do to support myself. Not that I had much choice, but I also wanted to find work that I found meaningful.

After my accident, I had experienced what many termed "Medical Intuitive Awareness." Lying on my couch with a migraine one afternoon, I suddenly "knew" my mom's friend had a serious thyroid problem. Embarrassed, I nevertheless insisted that she get it checked. She did, and the inquiry saved her life. The doctors had lost her blood work, and her thyroid medication had been poisoning her. This sort of "knowing" began to happen on a regular basis. Although I initially resisted my healing intuition, it seemed like a gift that I should share.

In the course of exploring what it meant "to be a healer," I took a Reiki class. Reiki (pronounced ray-key) is a gentle and natural system of healing. The Japanese "rei" means "universal," and "ki" means "life energy"—corresponding to *Chi* in the Chinese system of Qigong and acupuncture. Reiki, therefore, refers to the healing qualities of Universal Life Force energy. Another translation is "Divinely directed healing energy."

Besides learning how to perform Reiki on myself, I also learned how to give treatments to other people. I could not read, but Reiki—like all energy work—is more experiential than intellectual. My excessive TBI sensitivity actually *helped* me to detect subtle vibrations around other people and in myself.

I eventually became a Reiki Master Teacher. I believe the process of trying something entirely new—and mastering it—helped in my recovery. I had never even heard of Reiki before my accident. Four and a half years after TBI, I was teaching people how to teach. Playing a key role in others' spiritual and vocational transformations brought positive meaning to a difficult experience.

Now used in many hospital, clinic, and hospice settings, Reiki works on physical, mental, emotional, and spiritual levels. The gentle, noninvasive qualities of Reiki make it an effective therapy for people with extreme sensitivity to massage or chemicals. Reiki also provides non-drug pain relief.

- The International Association of Reiki Professional's website offers a way to locate a Reiki Practitioner or Teacher near you: *www.iarp.org.*

36. *Don't be afraid to pursue your dreams.*

On August 24, 2001, my parents' wedding anniversary, I met a man named Stephen. Immediately comfortable, I told him about my brain injury and my forfeited dreams of becoming an English professor. When I asked what he did, he replied, "I'm a writer." Intrigued, I asked about his projects, and we agreed to meet again.

When we reconnected, the talk again turned to writing and to my own frustrated plans to publish. I revealed my secret dream to write a book that bridged the gap between academia and pop culture. I had planned to bring together radically different disciplines. I had wanted to write a book popular enough that I could tour the country, perhaps even travel abroad on grants. I had wanted to make scholarship fun and palatable to the General Public.

As my appearance belied the severity of my injury, Stephen could not understand why I spoke of my dreams only in past tense. "Why not publish now?" he asked. I explained again that I could only spend about thirty minutes a day doing visual tasks. "So write poetry," he said.

The next time we met, I brought him three short poems. "These are definitely publishable," he asserted. "Really?" I asked. Stephen replied, "I guarantee that if you send these out, you'll get published by the end of the year." It was mid-October. "You can't guarantee that!" I laughed. "Send them out," he challenged, "You'll see."

Stephen gave me a *Writer's Market* book full of possible opportunities. When I complained that I would not be able to wade through all the print, he said, "You have good intuition. Why don't you intuit which places to send them?" His suggestions sounded just crazy enough to work, so I chose five markets and submitted the poems.

By the end of the year, two of my poems appeared in print. Two years later, I married Stephen.

Impossible things happen every day. If you have a long cherished dream, do not assume your health problems will prevent you from attaining it. You may need to go about it differently, but dreams do come true. The book you're reading now is proof.

Poppies and Sudden Snow Showers

When Dorothy sees the Emerald City, she becomes tremendously excited. Within moments, though, the Wicked Witch of the West finds a means to distract her: poppies. Out of nowhere, the sedating flowers appear, covering the very path that leads to the Wizard. Despite her enthusiasm, Dorothy grows so fatigued she needs a nap. Were it not for Glinda's magical snowstorm, Dorothy and her friends might have slept for days . . . or even years. This chapter offers ways to stay the course. It also increases your awareness of serendipity.

37. *Don't distract as you approach goals.*

Make a list of times in your life when you seemed on the brink of attaining a dream or long held goal. Did you miss any of these opportunities? If so, by what means did you miss them? How many months or years passed between each opportunity? Pay attention to any patterns.

Does some form of trauma always arrive when "everything seems perfect"? Consider the additional responsibilities that living your dreams, achieving your goals, or reaching full recovery would entail. List reasons you fear accepting this responsibility. Then find small steps you can take towards accepting more responsibility for who you really are.

Opportunities in life tend to cycle back in a recognizable pattern. Even The Yellow Brick Road begins with a spiral. Each time we miss a chance to move forward, the issue cycles back with more intensity. In the beginning, we receive an intuition or sense of what to do. If we ignore it, the next tap hits a little harder. After several taps, we receive whatever situation forces us to address the issue—usually our own worst nightmare.

Recognizing my brain injury as a major wakeup call encouraged me to get the message. I hated to imagine what the next "opportunity" might be. Responsibility became easier to embrace once I realized that I could only escape it through trauma, denial and disappointment.

38. Get plenty of sleep.

Before my injury, I was one of those lucky people who could get by on very little sleep. As long as I had a good six hours of rest, I could work, exercise, read a novel, cook, travel, shop, and socialize (all in one day) without feeling the onset of fatigue. Once in awhile, I indulged in a nap, but mostly for the novelty.

My high energy level frustrated and annoyed family members with more normal stamina. When visiting them, I often worked out for several hours just to be able to accommodate their pace. Although they feel guilty about it, each member of my family has privately told me that they found my diminished post-injury activity level much easier to bear.

Personally, I do not believe I will ever feel great about sleeping seven to ten hours a night. Personal feelings aside though, I can often predict the quality of a day based on how much sleep I get the night before. I have had to make peace with my need for extra shut-eye. Years of living with so much excess energy demanded I always be doing *something*. Sitting still induced anxiety and guilt because I judged myself by how much I accomplished in a day.

At first, having to devote an extra four or six hours to sleep seemed unfair. And lazy. Or depressed. Or spoiled. I could not accept that I simply needed rest. To me, going to bed before one o'clock and waking up after eleven held a stigma.

Embracing my extra sleep requirements was as difficult as accepting all the other changes after TBI. For years, whenever I imposed pre-injury standards on myself, I paid for it. So did everyone around me. Ancient symptoms reasserted themselves, and after two nights of sleep deprivation, I usually felt like the injury happened only yesterday. The harder I tried to bulldoze fatigue, the more dilapidated I became.

Eventually, a migraine, double vision, or the dreaded "spins" forced me to lie down. After a much-resisted nap, I could appreciate the irony: the longer I slept, the more I accomplished. I used to resent living like Rip Van Winkle, but REM became my fountain of youth. Without it, I felt too old to participate in life. On the bright side, having slept so many extra hours, I am now often mistaken for someone 10 years younger than my actual age!

Have trouble sleeping or staying asleep?

- Try Dr. Jeffrey Thompson's *Delta Sleep System* CD's. They'll knock you out (in a good way!).

39. Record your dreams.

Keeping track of nocturnal visions—on a notepad or tape recorder by your bed—can encourage insight and healing. In the midst of so much cognitive confusion, my dreams provided clarity often absent in waking life. With my perceptual problems, decision-making seemed a hopeless chore. Even questions of personal preference stumped me, because I could not discern how much of my "desires" stemmed only from the desire to avoid more pain.

In dreams, with their overblown mythic images and revealing juxtapositions, I could more easily recognize my true longings and emotions. A rich dream life also helped to compensate for the drudgery of days when I felt too dizzy to get off the couch. I began to sense a larger world—one in which I could still participate. Far richer and more beautiful than doctors' visits and court appearances, this dream world sustained me in an otherwise ugly stretch of life.

About two years after my TBI, I dreamt that my friend Kirt arrived out of nowhere and handed me seven miniature cheetahs. When I thanked him, Kirt replied, "You're welcome, but they're not cheetahs." I proudly walked them all on leashes, letting them part the way for me wherever we went. As I continued to thank Kirt for giving me such beautiful cheetahs, he became increasingly exasperated: "Damn it, Laura, they're not cheetahs!"

Wild cats often visited my sleep, but this dream seemed more significant because Kirt called me the following morning. It was the first time we had spoken in over six months, and he wanted to visit.

When I told the dream to a friend of mine who practiced Native American spirituality, she said, "Seven is the number of the sacred dream. Too bad they weren't jaguars. That would have been a very powerful dream. I don't know what cheetahs mean. I guess they're very fast." "Oh well," I sighed, thinking jaguars were only black—and ignoring Kirt's repeated message.

The following evening, I landed on a shamanism website and the first picture made me gasp. It looked exactly like the animals from my dream. A spotted jaguar.

This site quickly became a favorite of mine for dream interpretation and eventually for helping clients find their "animal guides." According to *http://www.geocities.com/~animalspirits/*, "Jaguar Wisdom Includes:

- Seeing the roads within chaos
- Understanding the patterns of chaos
- Moving without fear in the darkness

- Facilitating soul work
- Empowering oneself
- Moving in unknown places
- Shapeshifter
- Psychic sight"

Seven jaguars *did* seem like a powerful dream!

Eventually, I developed a dream relationship with one particular jaguar, who guided, comforted and protected me when my waking life became unbearable. Amidst Workers' Comp threats and accusations, financial insecurity, and an uncertain prognosis, I managed to remain quite calm. The jaguar's presence became such a part of my psyche that I felt nurtured despite the chaos. This secret and potent ally would make sure that I survived.

Those dreams, whatever their origin or meaning, allowed me to relax and heal.

40. Pray—with gratitude.

"That's the trouble. I can't make up my mind." The Scarecrow

After my injury, the part of my brain responsible for quick, rational decisions no longer worked. Choosing between Prego and Ragu at the grocery store once took over two hours. Eventually, I closed my eyes and grabbed a bottle off the shelf, just so I could leave the store.

Alarmed at the arduous, yet cavalier nature of my decision process, I knew I needed to find a better method. I had more important options than spaghetti sauce to deliberate.

Out of fear and desperation, I began to pray. I had prayed before my injury, but not with the same intensity or in the same way. I also had had less confidence in possible results. Instead of making random choices that might haunt me later, or getting a headache trying to navigate my options, I prayed for guidance.

About everything. Since everyday decisions about meals or clothes stressed me as much as bigger ones, I asked for help with these as well. To my surprise and relief, the "answers" came clearly and immediately. Whenever I slipped into a maelstrom of consideration, the rope of prayer pulled me to safety. As long as I listened to the guidance, I could navigate this world of confusion and debilitating pain.

Suddenly, I found myself making more authentic choices than I had pre-injury. I no longer second-guessed my decisions. I also developed a knack for serendipitously meeting the right people at exactly the right time. Whether from friend or treatment provider or lawyer, I found everything I needed just when I most needed it.

If situations seemed impossibly grim (and they often did), I remembered results of earlier prayers. Knowing I could consistently count on amazing outcomes saved me from despair. More than that, prayer opened my eyes to a bigger and more beautiful sense of order in this seemingly chaotic universe. Today, I feel more peace and joy than I ever felt pre-injury.

Besides providing guidance, prayer also helps to cultivate a sense of gratitude. In *Simple Abundance*, Sarah Ben Breathnach suggests giving thanks for five things each day. As she observes, the first few things may come slowly, but after three or four, you will probably have a hard time limiting yourself to five. That's the point—to make you aware of all the hidden blessings in your life.

Sometimes you may feel like your life already ended, and you got stuck picking up its pieces. If health problems robbed you of the life you knew, you might find it difficult to express gratitude for anything.

Do it anyway. Think of all the things that could have gone wrong but didn't—all the little miracles that went unnoticed.

Your health issues may remain, but how you deal with their presence in your life makes all the difference in the world. Recognize and appreciate the Grace in your life. You will see your blessings multiply.

"Surrender Dorothy"

When Dorothy and her friends first arrive in the Emerald City, they believe they have reached their destination. Joyfully, they prepare to meet the Wizard. Their dreams seem so close to realization that the Lion even dons a mock robe as King of the Jungle.

No one expects the reappearance of the Wicked Witch; no one anticipates that the most difficult part of the journey is about to begin. The message, "Surrender Dorothy," throws a shadow on the celebration and nearly defeats Dorothy and her friends. In order to receive their wishes, they must return with the Witch's broom. They must move outside their safe surroundings and face their biggest fears.

After everything you have risked, sacrificed and accomplished, another test seems categorically unfair. And yet, you will certainly face your toughest challenge when you get closest to your goal.

Mythological journeys always include a final test, and our myths reflect our lives. You are a hero. Strengthen your resolve to make it through your biggest struggle yet. Think of something you did today that you had never imagined you could do again. Now remember a personal miracle that you cannot explain away. Draw encouragement from your already "impossible" progress.

41. *Don't take it personally.*

When Workers' Comp hired a forensic psychologist to refute my claim, I took his report as a personal attack. Even though reading and writing resulted in severe migraines, I tried to defend my honor line by line.

Finally, my lawyer gave me this advice: "You seem to be expending a great deal of psychic energy trying to understand why someone would say such horrible things about you. It's really very simple. Your insurance company doesn't want to pay you. Will they lie, withhold information, and distort reports? Of course. I'm your lawyer. It is my job to defend you. It is your job to recover. Spend your energy doing that."

Brain injury litigation produced at least as much stress in my life as the TBI itself. My attorney was right. Insurance companies do not think of you as a person: you are a very expensive problem, which they want to eliminate. They do not care that your life has become unrecognizable. Nor do they regret the additional pain and suffering they cause you.

They *want* you to find this process stressful. They *want* you to give up, and if you won't *give* up, then they want you to *crack* up.

Do not give them the satisfaction. If your lawyer does not have all the facts, make him or her aware of any useful information. Then pray, sublimate, deny or forget—do whatever you can to let it go.

I drew. Long before I ever conceived of this book, I made *Wizard of Oz* Christmas cards for the two Workers' Comp women in charge of my case.

One cover depicted a house crushing the Wicked Witch of the East. Munchkins chimed, "Ding Dong . . . ." The other card showed her sister, melted in a pool of water underneath her hat.

The messages read essentially the same: on the front, "Christmas Wishes from Oz"; on the inside, "May you get all the blessings you deserve. Sincerely (*arrow pointing up*) Yours, Dorothy." Instead of Santa Claus, I drew and labeled a red devil, "Old Saint Nick," with the "Saint" crossed out.

I never mailed the cards, but the exercise released pent-up frustration. Finding an outlet for my anger allowed me to return more quickly to a compassionate perspective.

42. *Not everyone wants you to recover.*

This one sounds horrible, but accepting its truth can help you discern which advice to follow.

Sometimes family members and friends mean well, but they may unknowingly project their own fears and judgments onto your recovery attempts. Particularly if you have remained injured or ill for a long time, people have grown accustomed to viewing you as "the sick one" or the "one who needs our help." As you become more confident in your ability to make decisions, these people will challenge you. If you trust them, hear their advice, but balance it with your own sense of truth.

Rarely does "full recovery" mean a return to the pre-injury status quo.

What have you learned from your experience with brain injury or chronic illness? *What attitudes or activities make you feel whole and alive?* This information is vital to your healing.

43. Practice patience.

"For everything there is a season, and a time for every matter under heaven:

> a time to be born, and a time to die;
> a time to plant, and a time to pluck up what is planted;
> a time to kill, and a time to heal;
> a time to break down, and a time to build up;
> a time to weep, and a time to laugh;
> a time to mourn, and a time to dance;
> . . .
> a time to seek, and a time to lose;
> a time to keep, and a time to cast away;
> a time to rend, and a time to sew;
> a time to keep silence, and a time to speak;
> a time to love, and a time to hate;
> a time for war and a time for peace."

Ecclesiastes 3:1-9

If a brain injury does not teach you patience, then I don't know what will. Allowing recovery to unfold at its own pace is one of the toughest challenges of TBI—or any long term injury or illness. In my experience, patience comes slowly and only *with* experience.

Unlike the pre-injury world of deadlines, semesters, workdays and weekends, life with TBI sprawls onward like a desert landscape. Think of the pioneers crossing New Mexico in the 1800's: they did not know when it would rain; water was sparse; and civilization even sparser. They trudged onward, romanticizing the towns they had left behind or hopefully would find. But the journey through New Mexico must have tried their patience. If they wanted to survive the trip, they needed to carry their supplies. Traveling by wagon slowed them down, but it was the only way to go.

As a survivor, you travel with similar restrictions. You might hold a vision of what recovery looks like, but you cannot know when or in what condition you will arrive. In order to reach your destination, you need to survive the trek. Unfortunately, that means some habits, expectations, and coping mechanisms will remain for a while—even though they slow you down.

Trying to force yourself to the next plateau of health does not work, because change takes time. How many pioneers weighed down their wagons with a few keepsakes, which they could not bear to leave behind? You are in transition, too—moving towards an unexplored horizon, yet unwilling to part with all the old.

As you continue, you will lose your attachment to things that no longer serve you. For now, allow yourself to indulge in a little comfort and familiarity on the journey.

44. *Setbacks often precede big steps forward.*

Every once in a while—particularly during my 32 months of visual therapy—my symptoms would relax their constant harassing of me. Euphoric, I would tell all my friends and family that I had experienced a miraculous recovery. "That's great," they would say, "Just be careful."

"Careful?" I thought, "It's time to celebrate!"

I would then stretch the bounds of health as far as I thought I could. For some reason, I always needed to prove it to myself how far I'd come. Just when I thought I could count on this seemingly new level of wellness, a tsunami of fatigue would send me violently back to symptoms from several months or years ago.

Whenever a setback happened, I plunged into depression, calling the same friends and family members to inform them that I had not made a miraculous recovery. In fact, I had made no recovery at all.

People reminded me, "Laura, this always happens. Look how far you've come. You just overdid it. You *have* made progress. You're just tired."

"No," I said, "I feel like I did the first month after my injury. The room's spinning, and it hurts to open my eyes. I feel sick. I have to walk around the apartment with my eyes closed."

"Just sleep," they counseled, "You're transitioning. When you finish, your progress will solidify."

"But I *hate* sleeping!" I whined angrily, "I'm sleeping my life away." If I stooped to telling people what percentage of my 20's I had spent unconscious, they fell silent. What could they say? I felt like Sleeping Beauty, only not so beautiful, and my Prince Charming would have to be one hell of a healer to wake me up.

The people who spoke of my "transitioning," actually saw my situation more clearly than I did. As my behavioral optometrist explained, "We're trying to rebuild your visual system. Your brain compensated to some degree for all the damage. Unfortunately, the way your brain compensated causes all sorts of imbalances and cognitive problems. In order to rebuild your visual system, we need to destroy those compensations. In the period between destruction and new learning, you will go through some difficult times."

What an understatement! When my doctor warned me of recurring symptoms, I had not considered the toll a physical relapse might take on my emotions. Nor had I understood how much the physical changes in synapses would alter my cognitive processes.

During transitions, I felt volatile—like an electron that could not decide on which level to remain. In shifting levels, I changed what kind of person I was. I bounced around until I found something for cohesion—usually a new perspective on life.

Transitions lasted anywhere from three days to six weeks, recurring as often as my brain acquired a new skill. During that jumbled period of shifting synapses, my sense of identity dropped away, flared up as someone else, and eventually settled into something recognizable. Transitions were a natural part of getting well, but I loathed them.

Although I rarely remembered it in the midst of a transition, the wonderful thing about one was that it indicated progress. After days or weeks of dizziness, angst and a voracious appetite (sometimes I grew so tired of chewing that I resorted to blending two meals per day), the world became very still. I felt an ah-hah! lightning bolt in my mind, and my eyes snapped closer into alignment. As I resumed daily life, I invariably noticed that I could now perform a task that had been inconceivable pre-transition.

My longest and most traumatic transition resulted in a return of 3-D vision. Although I had described my TBI world as a "postcard," I had not realized the reason behind that description: I only saw in two dimensions. Everything looked flat and far away.

During this particular transition, I felt claustrophobic. I kept missing my mouth when I ate, because the food on the fork seemed several inches closer than it actually was. The walls pulsated as my brain tried to determine the real distance across the room. With the world suddenly closing in upon me, I grew irritated with people probably making only ordinary demands upon me.

It seemed as though everything and everyone was right in my face. "Back off!" I wanted to yell to the universe. "You're invading my space."

I eventually resigned myself to extended discomfort and asked people to give me a wider berth than usual. The transition's length encouraged even me to suspect a major improvement on the way. Because of the phantom movements of walls and floors, I knew it had something to do with spatial relations.

But I could not imagine how this reorganization would benefit my life. Only after my vision finished that first shift towards three dimensions, did I recognize how much more natural the world seemed, how much less effort it took to walk and to keep my balance. When objects finally revealed their volume, I also stopped running into them so often. According to my doctor, this shift from 2-D to 3-D vision marked a huge step forward in my healing.

Recovery from TBI does not occur in a linear fashion. It moves in fits and starts, setbacks and leaps forward. No one can give you a roadmap, because no such thing exists. As you jostle around uncontrollably, you are probably not the best judge of your current state of health. It helps to have friends and family who know your symptoms and who can recognize initial signs of fatigue or transition.

You might mistake a transition for a bad mood or relapse, thereby succumbing to depression. If you do not have anyone to help you through these times, consider talking to a psychologist, minister, or social worker. Whenever you find yourself discouraged, reviewing patterns like those mentioned in Hint #16 becomes particularly important. Seeing how a big step forward follows a setback can give you courage and stamina through the rough spots of recovery.

Melting the Wicked Witch

Remember your inner Wicked Witch? She's back with a vengeance. As you forge further along your spiritual path, your ego finds trickier ways to thwart your progress. This chapter suggests ways to transform attachments and expectations into opportunities for healing.

45. *Hold a funeral service for your "old self."*

Though it sounds funny or drastic, this type of ritual offers a cleansing and supportive way to move forward. On May 19, 1998, I lost the life I knew. Before my "funeral," I felt haunted by the ghost of my former self. I had lost my job, my doctoral scholarship and many of my friends, but old expectations and disappointments remained.

Like a spirit that could not rest in the afterlife until it experienced closure, I tormented myself with memories. If you spend the majority of your time contrasting the current you with the old you, then you probably need a metaphorical way to bury the outdated version of yourself.

As I reached new levels of cognitive improvement, I also struggled with the rapid changes in my personality and world-view. The brain injury itself had caused such a sudden identity crisis that I often clung to my now familiar self-definitions: "I have a brain injury; I am disabled; I cannot read; I cannot tolerate much stimulation."

Pain, confusion, and certain physical restrictions became the life I knew. Change—even in a positive direction—sometimes seemed traumatic and scary. Creating a small ceremony to honor where I had been helped provide the closure and courage I needed to move forward.

Depending on your inclination and imagination, you may wish to incorporate some of the following suggestions:

- Use the ritual for "Burial of the Dead" from the *Book of Common Prayer.*
- Paint a tombstone with the TBI date as your death date.
- Make a collage that memorializes whom you used to be.
- Write a eulogy or epitaph for your old self.
- Hold a wake with obliging friends and family members.
- Bury a box of photographs or poetry.
- Write or dictate the obituary for your former self.
- Burn symbols of things that you have outgrown or wish to change.
- Light a candle in honor of your new beginning.

As tempting as it sounds, I do not recommend burning all your medical records!

Tired of unpacking stacks of legal and medical documentation each time I moved, I decided to torch the entire mass at a Summer Solstice party in 2002. True to my continual expectation of miraculous healing, part of me expected instant recovery. Although I enjoyed watching flames engulf Workers' Comp correspondence and years of suffering, the process remained entirely symbolic.

Worse yet, I ended up needing copies of some medical reports as proof of lingering disabilities. I had to request these documents from doctors who had already copied my huge file numerous times for me—not to mention all the lawyers and insurance adjusters. My chagrin took something away from that daring act of conflagration.

If you decide to destroy something, make sure you can really live without it.

46. Forgive whoever caused your injury.

I felt sorrier for the woman who hit my car, than I did for myself. How would I feel if I had caused this much pain and suffering to another human being? From my deposition, she knew much of my anguish, but nothing of my spiritual and personal growth. I expected her sympathy.

When I heard about the woman's testimony in court, I felt shocked and betrayed. She answered, "I don't know" or "I don't remember" to 80% of my lawyer's questions. Then she outright lied.

I could not initially understand why she felt compelled to do so when her insurance policy would have more than covered my medical bills and economic loss. I later heard that her insurance company had implied her parents would lose their home if I won the lawsuit. The terrified woman thought she had to choose between honesty and ruining her family's life. I still feel sorry for her.

Justice does not end (or necessarily begin) with the American legal system. Can you really put a price tag on pain and suffering? If your experience ultimately leads you to live a more authentic and fulfilling life, then how does that factor into the equation?

Anger at the person who hit you or at their defense attorney will accomplish nothing. Life has a way of evening the score without our interference. Somewhere inside, they know what they did. If they are not already beating themselves up for it, then something else eventually will.

You will not recover fully until you can release your attachments to what you think is fair.

47. *Choose recovery AND financial security.*

If insurance refutes your claim, you might need to beg, borrow or barter for treatment.

I told potential providers about my financial situation and accepted any discounts they offered. I also borrowed $25,000 from my grandmother and loaned a physical therapist my car in exchange for sessions. In 2003, I went further into debt just so I could write this book. Partially disabled, I considered such actions an investment in my future ability to support myself.

Keep in mind that insurance companies and lawyers often scoff at so-called alternative medicine. If you seek a personal injury settlement, involvement in non-traditional treatments may hurt your claim. I decided I would rather recover as quickly as possible, than wait for a settlement that might not materialize.

Financially, I paid a hefty price for my choice because the defense succeeded in presenting my primary treatments as "snake oil." On the other hand, I healed, even though Western medicine offered no solutions. Make a decision and live with it. The process will empower you.

The following list details potentially helpful therapies that insurance companies and lawyers sometimes consider suspect:

- *Acupuncture*—now gaining recognition by some insurance companies and included as an option in some plans.
- *Behavioral or Neuro—Optometry*—not usually covered by insurance, but if the visual therapy is recommended by an ophthalmologist, neuropsychologist or physiatrist, insurance will sometimes cover a limited period of treatment.

  Some vocational rehabilitation programs and state programs for the blind and visually impaired will sponsor treatment that helps you recover enough to return to work. Neuro-optometric therapy is more difficult to find, but more obviously related to a TBI claim.

  For more information, see Dr. William Padula's essay in Appendix 1.

- *Chiropractic*—depending on your health problem, some insurance companies will pay for a set number of sessions, but usually not long after the acute stage of injury.
- *Counseling*—sometimes covered by insurance, if it seems related to your health complaint. *Beware that "confidentiality" is a relative term when it comes to insurance companies and lawsuits.* Even if your therapist

writes very brief notes, people will scrutinize them for ways to dismiss your claim as psychological.

Ironically, you might be better off treating with someone who has less education. Some minimally credentialed therapists are extremely effective, and courts will put less weight on their notes. Alternatives include talking to a priest, pastor, life coach, guru, or mentor.

Some churches also offer "Stephen Ministers," people from the congregation who walk with other members through life's unexpected challenges.

These alternatives are not "therapy," but you might reap more benefit from them in long run if you would remain guarded in traditional counseling sessions. Another bonus: some of these options are free, on a sliding scale, or "by donation."

- *CranioSacral Therapy*—not usually covered by insurance, but most practitioners hold degrees in other healing modalities. Your practitioner can sometimes bill for massage or physical therapy. For more information, see Hint #4.
- *Feldenkrais*—helps realign your posture for maximum ease and healing. It would depend upon the insurance company and credentials of the practitioner, but a growing body of research supports Feldenkrais therapy.
- *Herbal Remedies*—sometimes covered if recommended or administered by a licensed naturopath or physician.
- *Hypnosis*—with a referral from an M.D., insurance companies might cover a limited number of sessions. Be careful, though. You might want to pay for this one on your own, as it could be misconstrued. Your desire to try everything to get well rarely sits well with an insurance company. If you receive maximum benefit from hypnosis and the insurance company knows, then they may use it to prove your problems are entirely psychosomatic.
- *Nutritional Counseling*—sometimes covered if you and a physician can argue the case for nutrition's impact on your health complaint. Obviously, it would be easier to argue in the case of high blood pressure, heart attack, stroke, diabetes, or something typically recognized as influenced by diet.

Chronic Fatigue Syndrome and Multiple Chemical Sensitivities are increasingly being linked to "leaky gut syndrome." In fact, many experts believe that all diseases and conditions result in some degree from an unhealthy colon. Even if insurance will not cover it, you can often learn a great deal from one or two consultations with the right provider.

- ***Reiki***—works along the same meridian system as Acupuncture and Acupressure; however, Reiki's emphasis on spirituality and its lack of standardization and licensing makes Reiki a red flag for insurance companies and lawyers alike.

As a certified Reiki Master Teacher, I highly recommend Reiki's gentle healing ability, but I suggest you pay for it out of pocket or find a church or local Reiki Circle that donates its services to the community. Even more empowering, you can take a Reiki course and learn how to treat yourself. For more information on Reiki classes or treatments, please see: *www. internationalrenaissancecoaching.com* or *www.iarp.org.*

Note:

Originally, this hint read, *"Decide which is more important: recovery or financial stability."* The information ended at the last paragraph, because I could think of nothing more to share. For years, recovery seemed like an either/or scenario, with the implication that someone could not have both physical and financial healing. I wrote this book over a period of five years, though, and during that time, experience has taught me otherwise.

When I approached my 2002 personal injury trial, I could not imagine recovering both health AND finances. Part of me really did not want to win the $2.4 million my lawyer demanded because if I had won that much money for being injured I would have felt obligated to *stay* injured—for the rest of my life.

I had had private detectives on me for four years and I figured they would have followed me around forever, trying to prove insurance fraud. Even though I legitimately had "permanent brain damage," in my mind, winning a settlement of that magnitude precluded a miraculous recovery.

Oh, how I wanted that miraculous recovery! *In fact, I demanded it.* I said repeatedly, "Given the choice between $2.4 million and health, I choose health." Over and over again, I phrased this request, "If I win, I know I'll never recover. I choose recovery." (Unspoken implication: "Please, don't let me win.")

When I lost my personal injury trial—I got nothing because the defense found ways to exclude accident-related medical records from evidence—*everyone* freaked out. My dad told me I'd be homeless unless he supported me for the rest of my life, which neither of us wanted him to do. My mom resented all the trips to Independent Medical Evaluations, "the sick attempt to put a price on injury," and over a week of hotel costs in Putnam County, New York. Relatives contacted my family and chastised them for getting me "such poor legal representation, you *idiots!*" Well-meaning friends plunged into depression. My hotshot lawyer lamented needing to find a new career.

My loss had seriously rocked their world. I felt bad that everyone else felt sad, but personally, this was the most promising message I'd ever received about a full recovery.

I called my lawyer and told him that for three months I had had an entire monastery praying morning and night about my trial. I reminded him of all the spooky-weird coincidences in the courtroom, leading the defense attorney to hint about requesting a mistrial.

(The day my trial began, an independent organization had put up posters in the courthouse lobby describing "Shaken Baby Syndrome" and how a brain injury can happen even with seemingly mild accidents. A potential juror during jury selection spontaneously gave all the candidates a lecture on how it takes years to recover from even "mild" traumatic brain injury. Documents mysteriously resurfaced, which exactly supported my testimony. There was an earthquake.)

I told my lawyer it was "meant to be." Then, I called my friends and family and told them not to worry: I *would* recover.

Years later, when I had recovered, my dad mentioned losing the personal injury trial, to which I replied, "Yeah, but I *knew* I would get well." He asked me how I had known—since time had proven my faith correct. My answer surprised even me: "I knew I would recover because I *demanded* it. If I lost that trial, there was NO WAY I was staying injured. I didn't care what kind of miracle it required, that miracle was mine. I was not about to live without it."

My dad laughed and said, "Hmmm . . . that's so different than the way I think. My philosophy is, 'you live and then you die.'"

I suspect more people follow this philosophy than the one I expressed. I spent a couple of months congratulating myself: "Wow, that's so great that I could see another possibility, and that openness allowed me to get well against all odds."

Then I realized that *I* subscribed to the same limitations in a different form. Whereas my dad had envisioned an impossibility, I had envisioned an either/or scenario. The possibility of a full health recovery *and* full financial recovery did not exist in my current reality. I had accepted the idea that I would never equal or surpass my pre-injury income because I no longer wanted to work in sales. Insidiously, this limiting idea had put a cap on my aspirations, and so my annual income hovered about $37,000 below its pre-injury level.

It took effort to reframe my thoughts, and some courage to put my intuitive abilities on display, but I can happily say that I now make more money from more fulfilling work than I did pre-injury. If you recognize the *possibility* and commit to finding a way, so can you.

48. *Quit looking for shortcuts.*

In many ways, my pre-injury sales job seemed an appropriate career for me, because I was such a results driven person. "Give me a quota," I argued, "And I'll hit it. Dangle a bonus in front of me, and I'll reach it. Just don't ask me to write down how I spend my day. If I exceed your expectations, then why does it matter *how* I work?"

I resented having to track my progress. I thought people who talked about "process" only did so because they had not reached their goal. If someone worked ten hours a day to accomplish what I did in six, then I did not want to be punished for efficiency. Nor did I feel like sharing my shortcuts. If people knew how fast I worked, they might expect more from me.

I wanted people to underestimate me, so that bonuses remained easy and attainable. The idea of working hard just to say I had tried my best never occurred to me.

Even earning my Master's degree, I had found ways to minimize effort. Choosing incredibly creative paper topics allowed me to avoid the library. If no one had thought of a topic before, then there would be no articles to research. I churned out papers with a streak of insight and an edge of sarcasm. Most doubled as satires of academia.

Something in me—laziness, impatience, perfectionism—made the search for shortcuts automatic. If I skated through life quickly enough, I had no time to look at surroundings that might not meet my expectations. Unfortunately, I also missed the scenic overlooks.

The last time I remembered finding real satisfaction from anything was when I had written my college honors thesis. I had not been in such a hurry then. Nor had I written the paper in order to win the English Department's Whitfield Prize for best honors thesis. I had decided to write an honors thesis because I loved *Paradise Lost* and wanted to understand the poem on a deeper level.

Alchemy, the Apocryphal *Book of Tobit*, and Plato's *Symposium* had become the basis for "Milton's Phoenix: Raphael, Poetry and Transmutation in *Paradise Lost*," a 56-page paper that touched my heart. Those spiritual and intellectual discoveries had seemed far more important than the recognition I eventually received for winning the Whitfield Prize. I had thrown myself into the project and performed the work with love.

It strikes me as I now write that I not only relished the thesis process, but that the thesis itself was very much *about process*. Milton uses alchemy, digestion and sex as fitting metaphors for spiritual growth, rational thought, and creativity. In each case, *process* produces the result.

The tragedy of *Paradise Lost*—Original Sin—occurs primarily because Eve succumbs to the serpent's promise of a shortcut. She wants knowledge without the learning curve.

One could argue that this fall from Grace happens every time we cheat ourselves of an experience we need for growth. The resulting twinge of guilt disrupts our sense of wholeness and connection. It separates us from the Self, and we temporarily lose our way.

A pragmatic and impatient disposition forced me to learn the hard way that there are no shortcuts to recovery. Like alchemy, healing is a mysterious, yet sequential process. With the proper catalyst, it can occur almost instantaneously, but recovery requires certain elements in order to occur. Regardless of desire, we cannot skip steps and still manifest gold.

Although my TBI resulted in overt processing problems, issues with the *idea* of process had long preceded the injury. I had written my honors thesis without absorbing its message. Quite subtly, winning a prize began to overshadow the real value of the experience, and my motivation in life shifted from passion to calculated result.

This new focus on goal instead of on progressive steps robbed me of a sense of satisfaction. It was as though I stuffed myself with life, not bothering to chew or digest it. I derived little sustenance from projects, relationships or events, because I kept focusing on what else I could devour. Like someone with a hyperthyroid, I never felt full. Nor fulfilled.

A major blessing of TBI—one I still struggle to accept—has been the realization that life is not about how quickly we arrive nor how much effort we can avoid.

Just as protein and fat molecules are the hardest to digest but leave us feeling full, trauma and tragedy are the most difficult experiences to process, but they provide lasting nourishment and strength.

When we stop looking for a quick fix, we find true sustenance. We move from fast food to a five-course meal of ordered elegance. Appreciating such a feast takes time, but we leave satisfied.

The Wonderful Wizard of Oz

The Wizard isn't exactly what Dorothy and her friends expected. Toto unmasks him as a charlatan. And yet . . . he does manage to provide everyone with exactly what s/he needs. He just does so in some unexpected ways. In the bigger scheme of things, the Wizard lives up to his reputation, but only after people see the man behind the mask.

Perhaps one reason for the enduring popularity of the supernatural *Wizard of Oz* lies in the story's acceptance of the natural. On the Yellow Brick Road, no one needs to pretend. The friends accept each other as they are. They also accept change and surprises without bemoaning how things "should be."

The hints in this chapter ask you to recognize the "rightness" all around you. They also ask you to look inside yourself. Really look. Appreciate the natural you: see how beautiful and whole you already are.

49. Create a sacred space for yourself.

In the midst of overwhelming levels of stimulation, it helps to know that you can disappear into your own private haven of relaxation. When visiting people, let them know that you might need an escape route if their company or environment becomes too much for you.

Whether you live alone or with others, I strongly recommend that you find a comfortable place for quick retreats. The more this area soothes your senses, the better.

My first sacred space was a forest green, combed cotton couch with the perfect combination of softness and support. No matter what the weather outside, this couch remained cool, and when I rubbed my bare feet on it, I felt instant nurturing. Earplugs, and an ice bag over my eyes completed the cocoon, encouraging renewal.

Before the injury, I had sold cedar products to department stores and shoe manufacturers. Whenever I lay on the couch, I could smell faint traces of cedar that reminded me of palaces in Egypt.

In quiet, cool comfort, I allowed myself to drift across the centuries, forgetting florescent lights, police sirens and too much conversation. I could feel myself surrounded by a gentle breeze, inhaling all the scents from *Song of Solomon.* Thirty minutes to an hour later, I returned, but a taste of that journey remained.

Ideally, you will become your own sacred space. I used to joke that I had become a meditation expert because I lay around all day contemplating nothing. How funny to discover that my joke was somewhat true!

When I finally found some audio tapes on how to meditate, I had already tried most of the techniques on my own. Shamanic journeys, images of light, surrender to all-encompassing love—all these experiences had arisen of their own accord as I rested on the couch.

Only when I had recovered enough not to need such frequent isolation did I recognize how much I had come to enjoy the solitude.

If you think about it, neurological problems offer fertile ground for meditation and spiritual awakening. Some people spend their lives trying to escape a limited sense of self in hopes of moving beyond the ego. They become stuck in the everyday details that seem to form identity.

"Brain fog" results in a forcibly altered state of consciousness, which you can choose to deny, resent, observe, or embrace.

Instead of lamenting the disappearance of parts of your old self, you might want to consider the part of you that remains unchanged. This part, this Awareness, probably grows most apparent when the rest of you shuts down.

Next time you feel fragmented and "just can't hold it together anymore," stop trying.

Take a deep breath and notice yourself noticing. Find your center. Find your *real* sacred space.

50. *Listen to Pink Floyd's Dark Side of the Moon.*

Possibly the greatest rock album ever made, *Dark Side of the Moon* has touched the hearts and souls of millions. This album could also serve as a tour through the busyness of life before TBI, the trauma itself, and an eventual acceptance of what happened.

Track 4, "The Great Gig in the Sky," eerily combines a funereal wail with overtones of ecstasy. It is the closest rendition I have found—in any medium—of that initial euphoria, coupled with unspeakable pain. That song never fails to calm me while simultaneously provoking chills.

In the eighth track entitled, "Brain Damage," Roger Waters expresses the shared surreal experience of people who suffer an insult to the brain—whether through TBI, stroke, drug overdose, or chemical imbalance. In the final song, "Eclipse," Waters assures his listener that "everything under the sun is in tune / But the sun is eclipsed by the moon."*

You might not understand your situation or its timing, but order prevails nonetheless. Having a sense of this order can help you resist despair when things seem hopeless or impossible.

I listened to *Dark Side of the Moon* several times per day for the first four months of my injury, and songs from it still make me smile. Something about the music encouraged me to believe those lyrics. Wondering when or if I would ever recover, I'd suddenly sense a bigger order, which I did not understand or see, but which Roger Waters *assured* me did exist. Years later, I retrace my story line with awe and know that he was absolutely right!

Although Pink Floyd denies any intentional synchronicity, you can substitute *Dark Side of the Moon* for the *Wizard of Oz* soundtrack. To experience the phenomenon popularly known as *Dark Side of the Rainbow*, set your CD player to repeat the album continuously. Begin the CD after the black and white MGM lion roars for the third time.

I had heard about this coincidence for years but never tried it until after my injury. I figured I might as well take advantage of a naturally altered state of consciousness. The ability to appreciate such things helps balance the downsides of perceptual impairment.

---

*   Waters, Rogers. "Eclipse." Pink Floyd Music Publishers LTD., 1973.

51. *Look for the bigger picture.*

If you were directing a film about your life, where would you include your health problems? At the end? The middle? How about the beginning? Would you flash back to your early childhood? What key moments might you show to illustrate the movie's theme? Does your life have a theme?

Take some time to examine various angles you could use to tell your story. Have you always been the underdog, or would your screenplay show someone who fell hard but returned to the top?

Would you focus on external achievements or inner growth? Would the movie be a comedy or a drama? What would you like viewers to take away from it? A good time? A lesson? An inspirational story?

You cannot control everything that happens to you in life, but you can control your attitude and interpretation of events. Decide what kind of life you want to live. Then live as you would want to see it played upon the screen. Act boldly, vulnerably and under good direction. Become a star worthy of that Academy Award.

Recommended viewing:

- *The Wizard of Oz*
- *Chariots of Fire*
- *The Scent of a Woman*
- *Lost Horizon*
- *Fifty First Dates*
- *Sliding Doors*
- *The Butcher's Wife*
- *Still Breathing*
- *Mary Poppins*
- *The Enchanted Cottage*

52. *Be yourself.*

"One's real life is so often the life that one does not lead."
—Oscar Wilde

The great and innovative artist Henri Matisse did not start painting until he fell ill and lay bedridden for an entire year. Prior to his illness, Matisse held an administrative court job. Today the very name, "Matisse," has become synonymous with "artist," but it took a life threatening illness to reveal the essence of Henri.

Each major illness or injury offers a similar opportunity to uncover who you are. With so many layers of enculturation forcibly stripped away, you can more easily appreciate your core. Who are you without all the extras? Who are you without the narrative of your pre-trauma life?

When doctors said I would not recover, my life seemed to determine itself through the process of elimination. I could no longer read or work or drive; it seemed like I had no choices left. I eventually learned that even a world of such limited scope demanded *some* selection.

The injury removed career opportunities, but an array of everyday choices remained. Recognizing the inevitability of making decisions encouraged me to take responsibility. If I could not escape free will, then I might as well make the best of it.

My appreciation for literature had grown out of an original passion for creative writing—something I always loved but was afraid to pursue. It seemed too risky, too revealing, and too close to my heart. Academic writing afforded a steadier income and a distance between writer and reader that felt safer, less vulnerable.

The timing and severity of my injury guaranteed that I would not become an English professor, but I wondered if I really needed to give up everything I loved about literature.

In October 2001, I began writing poetry, which taxed my eyes less than prose. The exercise reignited my love of creative writing. On a dare, I submitted five poems for publication. It seemed such an unbelievable success to have recovered enough to write a poem that editors' judgments no longer frightened me.

A month later, I learned that a magazine wanted to publish two of my poems! Encouraged, I continued writing—to the small extent that my vision allowed. A year and countless migraines later, I finished an essay for an Animal Communication Writing Contest. To my surprise and delight, I won—and my essay later appeared in an anthology.

The success felt wonderful, but also challenged me. I had remained disabled for more than four and a half years. I still could not function on someone else's schedule or in a noisy or overly visual environment. I could barely read, and yet . . . I was winning contests, publishing my work. The "old me" would have fallen back on a regular job or academia, agreeing to write for fun. But the "new me" did not have that luxury.

I could wallow in discarded dreams, or I could try to make an impossible one come true. To do so, I needed a new, non-flickering monitor. I cashed in an IRA to pay for a top of the line laptop with a large LCD screen. I had never in my life bought a top of the line anything, but I knew I could not commit halfway.

In the past five years, I have published over twenty articles and essays, several poems, completed *If I Only Had a Brain Injury*, created and maintained two websites, grown a successful coaching, intuition and Reiki practice, written short stories, and begun work on two novels.

Choosing consciously has brought responsibility, but also an incredible sense of freedom and joy. For a few years, I wrote full time, a dream held long before I ever thought of graduate school. Ironically, I can finally read novels again, but I would rather write them. Despite—or perhaps because of—my enforced limitations, I have found ways to pursue my true passion. My worst nightmare has become a dream come true.

The majority of chronically ill or injured folks I encounter never desired to lead "normal" lives. Most felt odd before their health problems, and some accept debilitating symptoms as justification for an alternative lifestyle. Without turning a physical problem into a psychological one, it seems essential to recovery that people permit themselves to be *themselves*.

The Wizard of Oz embraces the unique dreams and vulnerabilities of each character. Drink deeply of this message! Life over the rainbow can bring greater joy, fulfillment and peace than you ever knew before.

Epilogue

"There's No Place Like Home"

As the Wizard waits to take her home in his hot air balloon, Dorothy realizes she must choose between retrieving Toto and her own return to Kansas. Chasing her dog, Dorothy loses a chance to travel with the Wizard, but Glinda arrives when the girl is truly ready to go home.

The Good Witch tells Dorothy that she always had the power to take herself back to Kansas but that she would not have believed so until this moment. Only the journey could teach Dorothy that whatever she seeks already lies within her. Until this epiphany, Dorothy looked outside herself. Now she recognizes that she holds everything she needs inside her heart.

Toto's escape provides Dorothy the chance to say farewell. Throughout the film, she calls her companions the "best friends in the world." In reality, the love, loyalty and support they offer each other provide the very healing they sought from the Wizard. He only brings recognition to what has already occurred.

As with Scarecrow's diploma, Tin Man's clock, and Lion's medal, the trip to Kansas opens the door to the next chapter of Dorothy's life. Scarecrow and friends will rule over Oz, while Dorothy brings her journey's Technicolor lessons to the Kansas gray.

If you have embraced your recovery as a spiritual or mythological journey, then you have probably joined other people on their own pilgrimages to self-discovery. Sustaining one another through your vulnerabilities and worst fears fosters great intimacy and camaraderie.

Because you have grown, you may have connected with people in a much deeper, soul-felt way than you ever did before. You might keep in touch with these friends forever, or you might only hold them in your heart. In order to move forward, sometimes we need to leave fellow travelers when shared paths diverge.

One of the great ironies and truths of *The Wizard of Oz* is that Dorothy finally gets her wish to go home, just when she realizes how much she loved the journey. In an avalanche of bittersweet emotion, she opens her eyes with gratitude.

She loves these friends, and she cannot imagine her life without this journey. Nor would she want to. Her fear and sorrows only accentuated joy, just as light and shadow form a picture.

When she bids farewell to Oz, Dorothy accepts the black with the white. And smiles.

She awakens.

Appendix 1

Glinda's Secrets:
A Special Section for Treatment Providers
Written by Other Treatment Providers

NEURO-OPTOMETRIC REHABILITATION OR "I FEEL DIZZY AND HAVE PROBLEMS WITH MY BALANCE. WHEN I READ, THE WORDS SEEM TO MOVE AND ARE SOMETIMES BLURRED. I FEEL EYE STRAIN AND SOMETIMES HAVE DOUBLE VISION, BUT MY EYE DOCTOR SAYS THAT MY EYES ARE FINE."

By William V. Padula, OD, FAAO, FNORA,
Founding President of the Neuro-Optometric
Rehabilitation Association, International

The quote in the title is often heard from those who have suffered a head injury, stroke, or other neurological event. People who have incurred these types of events often have difficulties that they may or may not relate to vision. If they do recognize vision problems, they often go see an eye doctor who tells them that there is nothing wrong with their eyes.

This is a correct statement for most eye doctors who simply look at the eyes and check whether or not the eyes are sending information to the brain. To understand how vision problems can cause these types of symptoms, we must understand that there is a difference between healthy eyes and how the brain processes visual information to match with other sensory motor information.

There are two visual processing centers; the focal and the ambient. The focal visual process transfers information from the eyes to the occipital cortex which is the main part of the brain involved in seeing details. This is the part of the visual system that relates to attention, concentration, and points of detail. The ambient visual process is related from the peripheral part of the eyes to the midbrain where information is matched with other sensory motor systems such as vestibular (balancing center in the ears), kinesthetic, and proprioceptive systems (muscle and joint sensory information).

The sensory motor systems are important for providing information for balance and movement. In order to maintain an upright and erect posture, the peripheral visual system must match with the sensory motor system for orientation about being upright and for ambulation (walking). Once this information is matched in the midbrain, it is sent back up to the higher seeing part of the brain (occipital cortex) so that the focal system does not only isolate on details.

Following a traumatic brain injury, cerebrovascular accident, multiple sclerosis, Lyme disease, etc., dysfunction will often be created between how the ambient spatial visual process matches information with the sensory motor system. In turn, this mismatch can cause problems with concepts of visual midline. Visual midline is an important component of the visual system where visual information is organized around the perceived center of a person's body when they are in an upright position.

With mismatch of ambient visual information, a Visual Midline Shift Syndrome can occur where the perceived visual midline becomes shifted to the left, right, forward, backward, or a combination. Once the midline shifts, the brain perceives the floor as being tilted which causes a person to lean toward the shift in midline. This can cause balance problems as well as dizziness.

The result of this mismatch in spatial information can cause the focal process to not be organized or grounded properly. In turn, the focal system begins to isolate on details. For example, if the focal system does not ground itself with ambient spatial information, a person will begin to isolate on individual letters as opposed to seeing the whole page when reading. Movement of the eyes then becomes projected on the details of the individual letters causing letters and words to seem to shift, move, and go in and out of focus. This has been termed Post Trauma Vision Syndrome.

Even though a person may have healthy eyes and no damage to the eyes from a trauma or other event, visual processing can be interfered with and cause the syndromes mentioned above. Normal ophthalmological and optometric examinations will often miss these visual processing disorders. The doctor may in finding that the eyes are healthy and the person can see relatively clearly, tell the individual that there is nothing wrong with their eyes.

There is a need to evaluate the visual processing system in a different way than just looking at the eyeballs and whether or not a person can see print on the distance or near chart. An optometrist specializing in neuro-optometric rehabilitation has the skills necessary to evaluate visual processing disorders following a neurological event that may relate to the types of symptoms mentioned above.

Balance problems can be treated through the use of specially prescribed yoked prisms. The prisms will shift the concept of visual midline back to a centered position and in many cases will demonstrate changes almost immediately. This can often be an effective means of treatment for Visual Midline Shift Syndrome.

Post Trauma Vision Syndrome can be analyzed through a neuro-optometric rehabilitation examination which may include a visual evoked potential analysis (brainwave study of the visual process). At the Padula Institute of Vision Rehabilitation in Guilford, Connecticut, we utilize the visual evoked potential (VEP) to specifically analyze the relationship of the focal and ambient visual processes and then test utilizing lens and

prism combinations. The results will often document the condition of Post
Trauma Vision Syndrome as well as demonstrate the improvement from
use of lenses, prisms, and binasal occlusion.

An individual who has suffered a neurological event and has symptoms
and characteristics similar to those mentioned above should seek services
from an optometrist practicing neuro-optometric rehabilitation. The
Padula Institute of Vision Rehabilitation serves people from around the
world who suffer from these types of difficulties and also attempts to find
doctors in more local geographic areas to support the needs of these
individuals over a long period of time.

Vision problems are quite common following a traumatic brain injury
or other neurological event. These vision problems are usually not related
to problems with the eyeballs themselves, but are instead due to visual
processing disorders that affect how the brain organizes eye alignment,
focus, balance, coordination, attention, and concentration.

An interesting statistic is that 70% of all of the sensory nerves in the
entire body come from the two eyes. Between the focal and the ambient
visual processes, 99% of the brain receives information in relationship to
the visual system. Primarily, the spatial ambient visual process is the key
component of the visual system for providing stability for balance and
movement as well as being related to higher cognitive function.

The rehabilitative journey of a person with a traumatic brain injury or
other neurological insult unfortunately often ends before the individual finds
or is referred to an optometrist practicing neuro-optometric rehabilitation.
However, this optometric specialty should be a part of the multi-disciplinary
team treating individuals with these types of difficulties.

www.padulainstitute.com
www.nora.cc

Interview with Karen Rupert, RN, CRRN
Nurse Manager
Inpatient Trauma Rehabilitation Unit
Harborview Medical Center in Seattle, Washington

How and when did you begin to work with TBI survivors?

When I graduated from school I had no idea what area of nursing to go into (we didn't learn much about Rehabilitation). I was offered and accepted a position on the Rehab unit at Harborview, and that was how it started. But it wasn't until I had a close family member suffer a very serious head injury that I found out what it was like from the "other side," and it really changed the way I viewed TBI patients.

Harborview Medical Center is recognized as one of the top trauma hospitals in the United States. In your opinion, what are some of the factors that make Harborview so effective in trauma rehabilitation?

I think the volume of trauma patients we see, the longevity of the program, the fact that Harborview is part of the University of Washington so we are able to access the newest treatments, all contribute. We truly have a "team" approach; that is patient focused.

From your day-to-day contact with TBI survivors, please share some observations to help treatment providers understand better the physical, mental and emotional challenges of their patients.

The thing to remember is that no two TBI patients are the same. They l bring with them all the issues they had before the injury. With our patients there are often problems with alcohol or drugs, coping abilities (family as well), psych histories, or learning disabilities. When setting up a treatment plan all these things need to be taken in to consideration.

What family dynamics unfold around survivors? Do you witness any patterns repeatedly? How does family affect the recovery process?

Whatever family dynamic was in place before the injury gets magnified after the injury. It places an incredible stress on the family. Even with minor injuries, the person they knew has changed. How the family adjusts to these changes is critical. The tendency is to treat the patient as a "child." Mothers/wives usually adjust more quickly fathers/husbands have a much more difficult time, they want the patients "back the way they were before."

How do creative pursuits affect recovery?

I think it gives them new ways to express themselves. We had Karaoke one evening and it was fun to see the patients, who were withdrawn and discouraged, join in. We try to find out what kinds of things they did before and help them get back into those pursuits.

In your experience, what qualities should treatment providers foster in their patients? In other words, how can the medical profession encourage and develop a more effective "healing attitude" in survivors?

Focus on their abilities not their disabilities.

Of the "miraculous" recoveries you've witnessed, are there any common denominators?

A strong will to succeed; the ability to move on in their lives; acceptance by family and friends of this "changed" person; access to necessary resources, especially financial resources. All of these play a part.

Please feel free to share anything else from your many years of service to survivors.

I recently had a patient, who has recovered from a severe TBI, come back to see me after 20 years. She told me how much she thinks about the people who cared for her and what an impact they had on her recovery. I think, as caregivers, we forget how much of what we do affects peoples' lives. Keeping a positive, calm and caring attitude goes a long way.

Changing the World One TTouch at a Time

By Robin Bernhard and Sandy Rakowitz

TTouch has been changing the course of therapeutic healing with animals and people around the world for over thirty years now.

This ground-breaking work, developed by pioneer, Linda Tellington-Jones, is being studied by Robin Bernhard, LCSW, a psychotherapist who owns and runs the Virginia Neurofeedback, Attachment and Trauma Center in Charlottesville, Jessica Eure, Med, Ed.S., a new counselor who specializes in neurofeedback with Bernhard at VNATC, and by Sandy Rakowitz, a practitioner of Energy Healing Medicine and TTouch, who owns and runs One Heart Healing Center for People and Animals, also in Charlottesville.

Both Bernhard and Rakowitz have over twenty years of experience in their areas of practice, and together, they are making headway in the use of this specialized touch to help with people who have suffered from brain injuries. Bernhard and Rakowitz would like to see Charlottesville become a center for TTouch research and training. Just last year, they did a study which showed exactly what they and others have been concluding all along—that this specialized work can improve brain function.

So, what exactly is TTouch and how does it work?

TTouch is a gentle non-invasive system of bodywork comprised of specialized circular touches, lifts and slides that promotes communication throughout all levels of one's being. Linda Tellington-Jones states that the intent of TTouch is to activate the healing potential of the body at the cellular level.

Last year in Scottsdale, Arizona, Bernhard and Rakowitz used an EEG to study the brains of volunteers applying these specialized TTouches to themselves. At first they weren't sure what they would find. They knew from earlier EEG studies done by Linda Tellington-Jones and Anna Wise in the 1980's that both horses and humans developed an "awakened mind" while experiencing TTouch.

Anna Wise describes the "awakened mind" as a specific activation of delta, theta, alpha, and beta brainwaves, and a particular kind of mental processing that enhances intuition, creativity and insight, that can only occur while the body is completely relaxed. Amazingly, TTouch simultaneously relaxes the body, helping to release muscle tension, aches and pains while activating the thinking mind so that new information is readily absorbed.

The effects of TTouch really do sound too good to be true, but a look at its track record proves its value. The method for horses, first developed in the 1970's, is known as TTEAM (Tellington TTouch Equine Awareness Method). In the 1980's, Tellington TTouch broadened to include the world of companion animals. The techniques deepen mutual trust, understanding and strengthen the human-animal bond. In addition, it has been introduced as an effective and valuable method to reduce stress in wildlife rehabilitation and to enhance the well-being of animals in zoos.

Linda Tellington-Jones is an internationally acclaimed authority on animal behavior, training and healing. TTouch practitioners all over the world utilize this system of touch, movement and body language to affect behavior, performance, and health, and to increase an animal's willingness and ability to learn in a painless and anxiety free environment. Tellington-Jones developed different touches to soothe and teach horses, whales, snakes, parrots, cats, dogs, chimpanzees, and many more.

You name it, she's TTouched it, and more often than not, she's gotten great results! TTouch works for all species, including humans. In fact, Linda Tellington-Jones will be here in Charlottesville offering a TTouch For You training retreat for humans in May 2008.

In the Arizona study, volunteers agreed to have a total of three EEG assessments to record the effects of TTouch. The first EEG established a baseline of brainwave activity for each person. The second EEG evaluated the effects of the circular TTouch called the Clouded Leopard TTouch, and the third EEG evaluated the effects another TTouch called the Heart Hug. All assessments were completed at one sitting through out a two-hour period. The practitioners performed the TTouches on themselves.

The baseline EEG of some volunteers showed brainwave patterns that were likely the result of horseback riding falls. Brainwave patterns are altered by injuries, and show different activation patterns than healthy tissue. Even so, the results of the study demonstrated that the Clouded Leopard and the Heart Hug TTouches helped to re-balance and normalize brainwave patterns for these individuals with prior head injury.

Over all, the TTouches also appeared to reduce the de-stabilizing effects of the areas suspected of brain injury. When an area of the brain is injured, EEGs may show spikes of activity, general over activity or suppression of activity, as the brain attempts to work in spite of the injury. Neurofeedback practitioners have been using brainwave biofeedback to improve the cognitive function of brain injury survivors for a number of years, and have found that brainwave patterns following injury are not so easy to change.

When the Arizona study suggested that both TTouches could change the chaotic, out-of-sync patterning typical of brain injuries, and bring them closer to a balanced state in which the brain could function more efficiently, both Bernhard and Rakowitz were elated.

And Rakowitz, having such familiarity with TTouch, immediately saw the potential for TTouch to improve the lives of those suffering from brain injuries. Only a few months after returning from Arizona, she put together another small pilot study for individuals with brain trauma and asked Bernhard and Eure to assist in the EEG assessments. The participants learned TTouches they could do for themselves to reduce the impact of many common symptoms associated with brain injury such as: problems with pain, mobility, motor function and coordination, concentration and memory.

People with head injuries often feel isolated by the invisible effects of the neurological difficulties, so each participant was asked to bring a helper who would learn the TTouches alongside the participant and help them to practice at home. This study is underway, and so far, there have been many exciting changes with pain reduction, improved mobility, focus, concentration and emotional well-being.

All of the promising results from both the Arizona study and the group for people with brain injuries have encouraged Bernhard, Eure and Rakowitz to continue additional TTouch and brainwave research with head trauma survivors. They are looking for grants to fund these projects. They thank Linda Tellington-Jones for her work; and Animal Ambassadors for donating funding for the statistical research software; and Jody Joy, owner of Living Mind, who has generously offered to help in the creation of multimedia materials to document the work.

*   *This exciting information has been derived from an informal pilot study. Because the statistical analysis has not yet been completed, we cannot be absolutely certain that the trends will prove to be as strong as suggested here.*

Sandy Rakowitz owns and operates *One Heart Healing Center* in Charlottesville, VA. Sandy weaves together 20 years of TTouch training and teaching with 12 years of practicing and teaching Energy Healing Medicine with people and animals to create an integrated approach to healing on the physical, emotional, mental and spiritual levels for people and animals. Sandy is a Certified *TTOUCH* Practitioner for Companion Animals, *TTEAM* Practitioner for Horses, *Centered Riding Instructor*, and *Brennan Healing Science Practitioner* for people. Sandy also integrates *Animal Communication*, the use of therapeutic-grade essential oils and flower essences. Individual sessions, long distance telephone consultations and workshops are offered in TTouch, Energy Healing Medicine, and Animal Communication. **(434) 973-8864** *www.onehearthealingcenter.com sandy@onehearthealingcenter.com*

Robin Bernhard, LCSW, MEd has been in practice since 1985, with an ongoing interest in the integration of the innovative treatments of EMDR, traditional Neurofeedback and LENS Neurofeedback. These, combined with individual or family therapy, dreamwork or sandtray work hasten healing for people suffering from various kinds of trauma. Her areas of specialization include: the neurobiology of attachment, dying, death and bereavement, life transitions, PTSD, creativity and performance enhancement. She has been a consultant to the Hospice of Western New York, the NYS Department of Social Services in Chautauqua County, Chautauqua County Head Start and the Charlottesville-Albemarle Mental Health Association. For EEG assessment information, please contact **Robin Bernhard or Jessica Eure** at *The Virginia Neurofeedback, Attachment and Trauma Center.* **434-979-4901** *robinbernhard@earthlink.net*

Jody Joy is an expert at assisting organizations to communicate information effectively in a variety of media. She may be found at **LivingMind.com**

Appendix 2

Aunty Em!:
A Special Section for Caregivers

Before Dana Reeve succumbed to lung cancer, she continued her own and Christopher Reeve's legacy of supporting people with spinal cord injuries. I received permission to include her letter as inspiration to other caregivers. The world will miss such a dedicated and loving woman, but how many lives she blessed while she was here!

A Message from Dana Reeve:

Hi—I'm here to talk about caregiving issues. I know that if you are a caregiver you are extremely busy. This message will take two minutes. After my husband Chris was injured, it became obvious that paralysis is a family issue. The family plays a critical and extremely demanding role in the lives of loved ones affected by disease or trauma.

Taking care of our families' physical, emotional, social and economic needs can be fulfilling and rewarding. But caregiving for a person who is paralyzed is a job we don't really expect to get, and one we seldom ask for. The job can come with a tremendous amount of heartache and frustration. According to the National Family Caregivers Association, caregivers suffer more depression and other stress-related ailments than the general population. It's easy to see why.

We mourn our loved one's loss of mobility and independence. We also mourn our own losses: we feel isolated, we have no personal time, we feel exhausted, overwhelmed. And we feel no one else understands the demands placed upon us.

But caregivers can find great strength and comfort in sharing their emotions and experiences with others. The Paralysis Resource Center (PRC) can help you locate one of the many caregiver support groups around the country. You will also find links to useful caregiver Web sites, and to organizations that offer respite services so that you can take good care of yourself, which is one of the cardinal rules of caregiving.

Always be mindful of your own unique qualities, and remember that maintaining your own good health is absolutely essential, to you and to your loved one. It is not a luxury. It is a necessity.

And guess what. You are not alone. You are extremely valuable. And you and your family can lead active, fulfilling lives despite the challenges of paralysis. Don't be embarrassed to ask for assistance—it is a sign of strength and an acknowledgment of your abilities and limitations.

Within the PRC Web site you will also find information on various conditions related to paralysis, and on many common areas of concern (bladder and bowel care, pain management, sexual health, skin care, spasticity, etc.).

The PRC also offers detailed information and referral on adaptive equipment and modifications that will make the caregiver's life easier (wheelchairs, seating and positioning systems, bath, kitchen and other home modifications, etc.).

Look within the PRC to locate information on insurance and Medicare reimbursement, and other topics related to the "system" of health care financing.

If you don't find what you need here on the Web site, you can always contact one of the PRC Information Specialists by email or by phone. These numbers are listed below. Or, you can set up a convenient time and a PRC Information Specialist will call you.

In a section of the PRC site called **Caregivers**, we've listed some online resources to help you in your caregiver tasks, to help you get some relief for yourself, and to give you the tools you need when hiring personal care attendants.

Good luck! Keep in touch! And, remember, you're not alone.

Best wishes,
Dana Reeve

www.paralysis.org or 1-800-539-7309

Reprinted with permission granted in 2005.

Interview with
Motivational Speaker and Author of 34 Books,
Kay Strom

As the author of A Caregiver's Survival Guide: How to Stay Healthy When Your Loved One is Sick, you seem to understand well the challenges and struggles of people whose loved ones are sick or injured. You spent ten years caring for your disabled first husband. Would you please explain his diagnosis and some of his symptoms?

Larry's condition developed so slowly, so insidiously. At first, it was just "odd behavior," things that were hard to pinpoint. Then he became frighteningly "absent-minded"—losing bank deposits, running red lights and stopping at green lights, lending our house key to casual acquaintances. By the time he was diagnosed with a rare genetic condition called *chorea acanthocytosis*—closely akin to Huntington's Disease—he was limping badly and dementia was obvious.

How did these symptoms initially reveal themselves? Did you or your husband deny their existence? At what point did it become clear that things might not return to "normal"?

Larry never did comprehend what was happening, which for him was a blessing. We returned home from England, our last vacation together as a family, to the ashes of our home that had burned to the ground while we were gone. Larry was excited about the adventure of getting new stuff, was eager to spend the insurance money on fun stuff even though we had lost everything, and only lamented a piece of wood from which he was "going to make something."

That's when I knew nothing would ever be the same. On the rare occasions when I saw him catch a glimpse of reality, it was very sad. One time we were in a store, Larry shuffling along beside me making the odd noises to which I had become so accustomed, and a terrified mother grabbed her little boy and pulled him away. Larry ignored them, but his eyes filled with tears.

Did your husband at times seem like a different person? If so, how did you reconcile your role as wife to the man you married and then to this "new man"? A sudden change in personality is perhaps one of the greatest challenges to relationships. What advice can you offer loved ones dealing with this challenge?

He became a completely different person. And certainly our roles changed drastically. I would suggest encouraging the loved one to express his feelings *(he's likely confused and frightened, it's difficult for him to admit he needs your help)*, help him stay connected *(no matter what, he still needs to feel that he's an important part of the family)*, allow the person to be as independent and in control as possible, and be attentive to his spiritual questions *("Why me?")*.

What, if any, patterns did you notice in your own emotions and health during this period? Have you observed similar patterns in other caregivers?

Oh, my, yes! Desperation, resignation, exhaustion. One time I was able to get out to a Christmas party for a couple of hours. I was standing by the fireplace when a woman I had only seen once before and met very casually stopped to soak in the fire's warmth and made the mistake of asking, "How are you?"

I opened my mouth and out poured all my bottled up fears and frustrations and desperation. I could see the panic in her eyes and knew she would escape the minute she could get a word in edgewise, so I purposely gasped a breath in the middle of a sentence and refused to pause between sentences so that she wouldn't be able to get away. That's how desperate I was!

A couple years after Larry died, I saw that woman again and apologized profusely for putting her in such an uncomfortable position. She was extremely kind and gracious. But she will never know what a Godsend she was to me!

www.kaystrom.com

The Flip Side: Becoming a Caregiver

By Laura Bruno

I decided to share my experiences in providing care during my husband Stephen's bout with Lyme Disease. As Dana Reeve acknowledged prior to her diagnosis and then death of lung cancer, "[M]aintaining your own good health is absolutely essential, to you and to your loved one. It is not a luxury. It is a necessity."

So *why* do so many caregivers develop depression, cancer or other life threatening illnesses?

Because it is HARD to acknowledge your own needs while someone you love continues to suffer! When I married Stephen, I had already worked, taught or volunteered in a healing capacity for several years, but at home, I remained the one who "needed extra care." Even after I had made a full recovery, we continued out of habit to place my health and comfort as a top priority.

Then Stephen began exhibiting many of the symptoms I had recently left behind: severe headaches, visual disturbances, short attention span, sensitivity to *everything*. He also developed what we would later recognize as "Lyme Rage." My formerly sweet, unconditionally compassionate, and laid-back husband suddenly struggled to tolerate anyone and anything.

(Lyme Rage is an actual term used by some psychiatrists and Lyme Disease patients. The term refers to the impatience, frustration, anger, and aggression that result from neurological manifestations of Lyme Disease. More and more psychiatrists continue to notice that some patients with "anger management issues" and other symptoms responded better to antibiotics than to psychotropic drugs.)

Stephen never became violent, but his personality changed. He grew extremely critical of everything in his life, particularly of me. Suddenly, everything I did irritated or infuriated him. I hated confrontation, particularly our increasingly intense arguments, so the focus of my day quickly became how to minimize Stephen's irritations.

I knew he had a headache, and I knew how awful visual disturbances could be, so my heart went out to him. But his triggers increased daily: I could not possibly keep pace with his rapidly lowering threshold for stimulation or risk.

He had always been so kind, clear, strong, and convincing that for a time I really believed him that *I* was the one who had changed. A dark cloud closed around my life. This man, whom I deeply loved, with whom I had always shared everything, suddenly became someone whose words slashed my heart. On top of that, I could no longer access my best friend with whom to process the terrifying and sorrowful changes in our marriage.

One insomniac night, while sobbing on the couch for guidance, I realized that Stephen was in fact extremely ill. He had not been himself for months, and as I stopped blaming myself, I could see with clarity that he had something physically wrong with him.

His list of symptoms included chest tenderness and joint pain, along with the neurological issues. The problems had all begun around the same time—after he had had a strange rash appear and caught the "flu." As soon as I realized that I had not caused all the problems in my husband's life, I managed to get him proper treatment, both through the V.A. Medical system and through herbal and dietary supplements.

In that moment on the couch I recognized just how devastating a loved one's illness or injury can be to someone else—particularly when the ill or injured person *looks* exactly the same as before.

The experience of nursing my husband through Lyme Disease has taught me how difficult maintaining a caregiver's own sanity and sanctity can be. For months, I focused entirely on Stephen, allowing my yoga practice to take a back seat to his needs. Although vegetarian, I cooked meat constantly, trying to find some kind of food he might enjoy. I spent my former meditation time conjuring ways to give him fleeting moments of pleasure to distract him from his pain.

I repeatedly injured my neck, elbow, thumb and shoulder carrying far too heavy bags home from grocery stores, just so he would not need to get out of bed to drive me there. Despite Stephen's offers to drive me, I fought to keep walking. Those walks to and from the store constituted my only guilt-free "me" time each week.

After about eight months of failing to heal or comfort Stephen, I burned out. I accepted that perhaps I had been miraculously healed from my injury just to serve my husband's needs so he could continue working, but I felt little joy in life. Stephen had stood by me while I recovered, and so I would stand by him. Inside, though, my soul wept. I cried continually within myself, but I felt selfish letting Stephen know how much I suffered. He had his own problems.

Finally, I could no longer contain my sorrow. Tears spilled into the sink as I washed dishes. I sobbed in the shower. If it rained three days in a row, I wanted to die. One day, I suggested Stephen not eat because I was too tired to make his lunch. *Something needed to change!* I could not help him while I remained in such a state, and my depression dragged him down as well.

Stephen insisted we make a major shift. We moved from the Oregon Coast to a sunnier climate in a city near all the things we both hold dear: nature, mountains, lakes, rivers, plus my favorite vegetarian restaurant. Stephen accepted that my herbal protocol really did improve his symptoms and life as long as he regularly took the "medicine." He recognized that he needed to try his best to recover for me as well as for himself, and I stopped spending all my energy urging him to improve.

Stephen continues to pursue his passion of photography, and I started writing again, expanded my Intuitive and Reiki businesses and completely took over his Life Coaching practice.

I began regular yoga sessions and started meditating again. I sometimes follow a guided meditation CD by Yogiraj Alan Finger, called "Life Enhancing Meditations." I used to meditate without using a CD, but with so many pressing tasks, I find the guidance helpful. I don't have to work here: someone's helping *me*. I also started practicing Reiki on myself again—another thing I had become "too busy" to do as a caregiver.

Having those 20-60 minutes per day has made all the difference in my attitude, energy and compassion. I know I can return to a place of peace, and I know that the day's "doing" is nowhere near as important as simply "being." I remain present for Stephen and all my clients, and I no longer feel too tired to make his lunch! I feel joy on a daily, often continual basis, and this joy spills over into Stephen's life.

In returning to yoga, I rediscovered my love of Sanskrit—the most ancient Indo-European language from which most languages began. Something about listening to or singing ancient syllables calls me back to center and lets me live from a place of joy. Sanskrit "works" for me because it sounds primal and mysterious, and because it transcends my rational mind. I don't know what many of the words mean, but my body, emotions and spirit respond as though they do.

Stephen and I also found the healing mantras highly effective, particularly something known as the Ra Ma Da Sa mantra. It goes like this: "Ra Ma Da Sa, Sa Say So Hung." I used to sing it inside whenever I felt sad, or if Stephen's symptoms acted up, I "sang" the notes silently to him. It's both calming and healing, and the vibrations can actually transform a mood or pain. For a beautiful musical rendition, you can listen to the "Ra Ma Da Sa" CD by Gurunam, which offers this mantra set to Johann Pachebel's Canon in D.

Perhaps I had just been under way too much stress for far too long and the Sanskrit brought a fresher prayer venue. During my own recovery, I had found tremendous peace listening to the Psalms or saying Alcoholics Anonymous' famous Serenity Prayer. I memorized and often quoted The Prayer of St. Francis:

"Lord, make me an instrument of your peace.
Where there is hatred, let me sow love.
Where there is injury, pardon;
Where there is discord, union;
Where there is doubt, faith;
Where there is despair, hope;
Where there is darkness, light;
Where there is sadness, joy.

Grant that we may not so much seek
To be consoled as to console;
To be understood as to understand;
To be loved as to love.

For it is in giving that we receive;
It is in pardoning that we are pardoned;
And it is in dying that we are born to eternal life."

I still agree with the idea of surrender in this prayer, but having spent time as the caregiver for a spouse, I now understand how important it is to *receive* as well as give.

However you decide to nurture your own needs as a caregiver, *please,* find and practice something that brings you joy. Even if you take only a few minutes to pray each morning. Or to exercise. Find a moment in the afternoon to listen to your breath. Do something wonderful for yourself!

Your soul and your loved ones will thank you.

From the Wife of a Brain Cancer Patient . . .

By Stephanie Jellison

My husband Mike had an episode that led to the discovery of a high-grade tumor in the right frontal lobe of his brain. I want to discuss some of what we have experienced with the associated realizations. Although Mike is the one that had the brain surgery, this is definitely a "we" experience. The impact has been significant for both of us. Mike's treatment to date has included neurosurgery, radiation, chemotherapy, and gamma knife.

The storm that blew up has been a whopper. After surgery, Mike lost of the ability to move his left side from head to toes. He had to learn how to move again in spite of permanent weakness on the left side of the body and a decline in energy, vigor, strength, and heartiness.

There have also been many less apparent differences, but the impact of these changes has caused alterations to all aspects of our lives. Mike's memory, thinking, emotions—in fact his personality is different. He recognizes some of the changes—attention and concentration; learning and short-term memory; as well as problem solving and judgment.

Although directly impacted I am still an observer. So, I try to discern if it is a symptom that can be treated like a headache, vision problems or fatigue, or if Mike is suffering due to changes to his general cognitive abilities.

The care and treatments he has received from the medical community have all been focused on survival. Although we realize that "surviving" is crucial, we have come to deeply appreciate that "living" is important as well.

"I want to go home" was Dorothy's cry, and both Mike & I can relate to that plea. But the fact is that our reality is different, in some ways very different—home is not what or where it was in Kansas anymore. In fact, I have had to accept that I am not the same person I was before this happened and that I am now living in a foreign land.

Accepting this truth is a challenge. The changes to Mike's health and abilities have caused everything else to shift. Even our sense of reality is altered. Most of the changes are unending and our world will never be the same. Often the recognition of the loss or change has been a challenge in itself increasing Mike's distress.

I heartily recommend for anyone facing these kinds of changes that you avoid a preoccupation with what is lost. I try to view this as an opportunity for me to learn acceptance of "what is" just "is."

Since Mike is sensitive to the fact that there have been changes, I've learned not to overtly identify changes and to quit saying "well, you used to . . ." I've learned to be ready to repeat information over and over—but to avoid saying that it is a repeat because of the hurtful effect.

Mike and I are fortunate and there are many family members and friends that want to be in the know. Unfortunately, I have had very little energy and repeating what we heard from doctor visits and test results again and again was exhausting. Since the task of reporting fell to me, I realized early on that one-by-one conversations were not really doable. I knew that to endure I must find a good communication methodology.

Since the vast majority of our family and friends have email, my solution was to create a "Mike's Updates" address list. After each major event, appointment, major test or round of chemo I create one letter and send it to the group. If someone came and asked about Mike and Mike was willing to share the information with the individual, I'd offer to add them to the list.

I still had two calls that were required—his father and step-mom and his mother, but it was such an improvement over fielding 10-15 calls. For when the information was too sensitive, I created a phone tree and tried hard to limit the number of branches attached to the trunk. There may have been a few hurt feelings, but I believe that my primary obligation is to reserve my energy for Mike.

Mike has been left with persistent weakness to his left side, the subsequent tremors, and his loss of balance. The loss of physical strength and agility has been hard for Mike. It has limited action in all aspects including the hobbies that we have so enjoyed. Massage has been very helpful both during Mike's relearning how to use his left side and to offset the exhaustion of muscles that are not firing as well as they did pre-surgery.

Another big help was finding him some aids to independence. Unfortunately our insurance did not cover them but these two have been worth every penny—(1) anchored poles next to the bed and the couch that Mike can use to pull himself up; (2) toilet rails that assist in steadying himself down as well as getting up.

If you can be genuine, I recommend that you praise the effort being made. For Mike the effort to perform some everyday life tasks is now Herculean, I do my best to acknowledge that work rather than begrudging what he can't do anymore.

This has forced me to take stock of how much he did prior to surgery and how much I took it for granted. I have learned how to assist in transfers so I don't get injured. And once we were through with the hospitalization and rehab, I made sure that I scheduled massages for my health and well-being. I realize that I must protect myself so that I can be there for Mike.

About all those chores and tasks that cannot be done by Mike: I realize that absolutely everything takes more energy than it used to, so, I have identified what I am willing to let go of *or* accept at a lesser level *or* get help with. If you have family who is willing to help, this is an area where they could really be an asset.

If you are like us, most of your family is not at hand so you may have to hire help to do some of the work. This has been another financial challenge, but making this effort has helped me stay focused and reduced my falling back into the "I just want to go home" tantrums.

Mike used to be a man of multiple stimuli. In years past he would be at the computer programming, have the TV on, his iPod going and possibly be talking with someone on the phone. Now communication is a challenge. Both inbound and out bound.

Inbound: I find that Mike is less able to understand spoken language. I started seeing evidence that this was a permanent change rather than a temporary result of treatment because he was confused during conversations or while trying to watch TV or movies. We also noticed that new information is more difficult to learn and remember. Mike has had to learn to give himself more time to absorb new information and to take notes and refer to them to assist in remembering.

Since he never had to do this in the past, it hasn't come easy. A big help for inbound entertainment was purchasing a TV with closed caption functionality. Combining the visual and the auditory helped immensely. Also, Mike needs to be positioned in a conversation where he can directly see the speaker.

Regarding outbound communications, Mike has more difficulty expressing himself especially difficulty is word fluency or word-finding. It is as if the word he wants is on the "tip of his tongue" but he is unable to retrieve the word. Bottom line is that this has been one of my opportunities for learning patience and not jumping in to fill in the blanks.

Mike does not make decisions as quickly or have the same flexibility in thinking. My first response was to just make decisions when he did not respond. As you might guess, that was a very unpopular methodology. It was not unreasonable that a 42-year old man did not want to relinquish control. So, I have learned to change the time schedule for decision making.

Rather than expecting an answer, I pose the question and define the time by which I need to have an answer. As an example, when his brother is coming to town, I ask if he has any preferences for menu and tell him when I will be going shopping for the event. I bring it up again the day before I need to shop. Then I ask for a decision before I go shopping.

Lions and tigers and bears may be recognizable, but many of our "oh my" experiences have been around changes that Mike does not really see. It is as if he does not remember what he was like before. Those closest to

Mike can tell you that he now likes different foods and different colors—he even reacts differently to smells and sounds.

He has even become extremely texture sensitive. I fondly call it his princess and the pea phenomenon. Although in years past Mike would not have noticed, folds in sheets or grain of sand on the tub floor are now very uncomfortable. This requires extra effort to provide him a comfortable environment.

Following the Yellow Brick Road this last year has been a challenge that I could not have imagined. We focus on solving the issues that confront us, blessed with a great love that has become our haven in this foreign land. I continue to hope that we will get home all right.

Interview with a Spiritual Director:
Rev. Daniel Prechtel of Lamb & Lion Ministries

Even non-religious people turn to prayer when faced with crisis, and there are times in the recovery process when all a caregiver can do is pray. As a trained Spiritual Director, would you please share some ways in which prayer can help in times of struggle?

Prayer can both *connect* and *detach* us in healthy ways in times when we experience struggle. In prayer, we bring our concerns and desires for ourselves, or for others, to the divine mystery as we understand this mystery from our spiritual tradition and our experience.

Words or images may be used, but the prayer might be wordless and imageless. We'll talk more about that later. For some it is an aligning (or the desire to align) our deepest self with the Holy One, who is within and beyond us. For others it is a communication or offering to the Presence. So prayer may connect us with the deepest dimension of our self, and with God, and with others.

But prayer also helps us detach in healthy ways. It helps us to acknowledge our limits while giving us hope that we can offer our concerns to that which is "beyond" us. We don't need to carry the responsibility for the outcome of our concerns alone. The old Twelve Step slogan, "Let go and let God" is quite appropriate to times of struggle and crisis.

In the Christian spiritual tradition, with which I am most familiar, we can speak of God's grace being active beyond as well as within our abilities. Prayer is a way of giving our "consent" to God's desire and ability to go about the gracious work of healing.

Have you ever witnessed prayer accomplishing what actions could not?

Prayer *is* action. There are times when prayer is the only action we can do, and other times when it is an offering we make alongside other actions. Healing can happen through prayer. Sometimes the healing is physical, sometimes it brings spiritual and emotional strength and healing, and sometimes it opens up new and unexpected possibilities and capacities. I have witnessed prayer accomplish all of that. God can be very creative with our prayers.

If someone feels like s/he has depleted herself to the point where all s/he can offer are prayers, should s/he feel guilty? Why or why not? In your experience, how does guilt play itself out in our spiritual and emotional lives?

Guilt can be a red flag that something is out of order. I feel like I've let this person down—or I've let myself down—or I've let God down—by something I've done or haven't done. In the situation you describe, the person feels depleted and has nothing left to offer but prayers. Should she feel guilty?

I can't judge that. But she might or might not feel guilty. She might feel guilty because she has allowed herself to be depleted. Or she might not because she felt she has done everything she could possibly do. However, if the person *does* feel guilty it is important to respond to the guilt in a healthy way.

Unrelieved guilt can increase anxiety, undermine self-worth, and erode the spiritual and emotional level of relationships with others and God. But when guilt has been directly and lovingly addressed, these can be occasions of transforming grace and forgiveness and reconciliation. S/he might talk to a trusted person about her feeling to help her decide what an appropriate way to respond is.

Spiritual guides, pastors, or counselors can be confidential sources of help. Dealing appropriately with guilt might result in a change in behavior, or an acceptance of limits, or a new way of understanding the expectations in the relationship. Some faith traditions have rituals of confession and forgiveness to help deal with matters of sin and guilt.

When people hear the word, "prayer," they often think of a bedside recap or list of requests. Mystics teach us that prayer can be more than narrative. Would you please describe some different styles of prayer? What are some techniques for these styles of prayer? To what types of people or circumstances might each style appeal?

I like to use a fourfold spiritual path model that some authors (especially Corinne Ware) refer to as "head path," "heart path," "mystic path," and "kingdom path." We have each of these capacities within us but tend to have one or two "paths" that we habitually use.

The *head* path might include reciting written prayers and litanies throughout the ages and other narrative styles of praying, and meditating on the meaning of scripture passages. These prayer forms are typically thoughtful and orderly. Praying the "Hours" in some form provides some people with a way of dedicating themselves to God throughout the day.

The *heart* path might include expressive and spontaneous forms of prayer, Ignatian-style imaginative meditation with scripture, guided imagery prayer and meditation, ritual healing prayers, the arts as prayer practices, or sacred movement and dance and chant. Gospel hymns or renewal songs are forms of prayer on this path. A parishioner who was a jazz pianist learned that he best prayed through his fingers on the keyboard!

The *mystic* path touches on holy mystery. Here the emphasis is in silently and simply being with the God that is beyond our comprehension but is already connected with us in love. Centering prayer and other forms of contemplation mark this path. Often the prayer might be wordless, or just one centering word, or be a very simple chant, or consist of sitting silently with an icon or candle flame or other sacred symbol that helps us be attentive to the unseen Presence.

The *kingdom* path focuses our attention on the connection between the spiritual and the physical and moral needs of the world. This draws on the Hebrew prophetic tradition of justice-making and ethical imperatives. It calls us to follow in the footsteps of Sojourner Truth, Mohandas Gandhi, Martin Luther King Jr., Dorothy Day, and others who work for justice and reconciliation in our world.

All of these spiritual dimensions are within us. At different times in our lives we might find that one or another path is more fitting to our circumstances. In times of trauma, we sometimes find ourselves unable to pray in ways we could in the past. When things are unclear and dark and forces seem overwhelming it might be a time to practice some of the simplicity of the mystic path.

If words don't come, perhaps we are invited to simply sit with an open heart and invite the Holy Mystery to be with us in whatever way God will. Or maybe we are invited into the heart path and pray by drawing a picture of our pain and hope, or use a journal to have a dialogue with our inner Wise One, or imagine making a journey to the Christ Spirit and being soaked in healing light.

Survivors' loved ones sometimes experience potent dreams or "funny feelings" shortly before their loved one's injury or illness begins. How might such synchronicities (meaningful coincidences) bring comfort or peace to them as traumatic events unfold?

On one of the deepest levels of life, we are all connected—we live in a web or network of relationships. The depth psychologist Carl Jung called it the personal collective unconscious. A Christian understanding might see this connecting as an aspect of the work of the Holy Spirit and the communion of the saints.

Western emphasis on individualism leans too much on our separateness and fails to appreciate the collective realm of experience. An intuitive "knowing" from that level through dream images or feelings might be experienced as a consoling assurance that the loved one is truly connected at a deep level of reality that transcends space.

Why do dreams speak to us so strongly during times of change? How can people draw upon their dreams for healing, comfort and inspiration? Are there any traditions of caregivers using dream work to help sick or injured loved ones?

Dreams are an important window to our inner reality that reveals aspects of our lives that might be filtered out in our waking state and also may give hints at directions for us to take toward greater growth and wholeness. The Rev. Jeremy Taylor, one current writer on dream work, contends that *all* dreams come to us for the purpose of greater healing and wholeness. However, dreams speak to us in symbolic language and it can be tricky to learn that language. Symbols can have many meanings, and can speak on multiple levels—ranging from the individual to interpersonal to societal to global concerns.

During times of change and trauma the unconscious content of our lives are likely to be nearer to the surface, so to speak, and can come to us with greater urgency and clarity. These are times when our sensitivity is heightened and are feelings are sharper.

We might think of one aspect of dream imagery as pictures of our feelings. In times of change our inner wisdom, which may be speaking to us through our dreams, is telling us to pay attention! The inner wisdom has something to say to the dreamer.

In ancient Greece, sick people would make pilgrimages to healing temples where the god of healing, Asclepius, would come in a dream to give directions for cure or greater health. That capacity for receiving inner directions toward greater health is still with us. Psychotherapy has drawn on this ability for profound inner healing and relationship building, but we need not be limited to therapeutic resources alone.

In many cultures it is not uncommon to share dreams with friends and loved ones, and sometimes with the spiritual guides, to gain and share insight. Caregivers might form a dream-valuing community for mutual support, hearing each others dreams, and assisting each other in exploring the path of healing for themselves and their sick or injured loved ones.

The sick or injured persons shouldn't be kept out of the circle of dream-valuing if they are capable of communicating their dreams and hearing yours. In the dream sharing, explore the question: what is this dream asking me/us to pay attention to for greater healing and wholeness?

What kinds of things can people do to deepen or intensify their dreams? Can dreams support intentions?

The more you value dreams—your own and others' dreams—the greater will be your ability to remember, deepen, and intensify your dreams. Keeping a dream journal, making entries in the morning when you awaken, will develop your dreaming recall ability and will increase the clarity of your dreams. Sharing dreams with other people will help cultivate the capacity for being a creative dreamer and help you be in touch with your inner wisdom.

You can pray for dream insights. The ancient practice of "incubation" of dreams is something you can do—as you think of a particular intention throughout the day, tell yourself that you will soon have dream that will help illuminate that intention. Do the same thing immediately before you go to sleep. This incubation practice will eventually induce a dream on the subject if you keep at it.

Often we unintentionally induce dreams because we are steeped in a situation in our waking and will revisit it in our dream state, but we can intentionally induce them by applying the incubation technique.

What do various religious traditions tell us about the idea of selfless service? How might caregivers deepen their own experience of life through the process of caring for a sick or injured loved one? Is there a patron saint of caregiving?

I think that every major faith tradition values selfless service. Islam, Judaism, Hindu, Buddhist, and Christian values all support being compassionate (*com*=be with, *passion*=suffering). Being compassionate doesn't mean we should ignore our own needs (for we need to be compassionate with ourselves too), but it calls us to go beyond our needs alone and look to those of others. The experience of caregiving helps us go deeper into the heart of our humanity.

We are interdependent with the rest of creation and can never be fully alive by ourselves apart from the rest of life. All of us need help in various ways throughout our life—and to live deeply acknowledges the mutual giving and receiving that is at the heart of existence. A Muslim calls upon Allah, the Merciful and Compassionate One. Jesus taught his disciples to lead by being servants to each other and spoke of his Father as loving and knowing our needs.

In various ways, religious traditions call us to be compassionate people in the service of those in special need—it is the kind of love that is at the center of the cosmos.

Is there a patron saint of caregiving? Probably many patron saints. Certainly, Mother Teresa of Calcutta stands out as a possible candidate. I expect that in any religious tradition there are exemplary people that would qualify.

For example, in my Anglican tradition we have a feast day for Elizabeth, Princess of Hungary, who died in 1231, who provides a strong testament to selfless service and compassion. She used her dowry for the poor and the sick. During a famine and epidemic in 1226, she sold her jewels and established a hospital where she cared for the sick and the poor. She opened the royal granaries to assist those in need.

After her husband died, she became one of the first Third Order Franciscans and lived in self-denial, caring for the sick and needy. She and Louis of France share the title of patron of the Third Order of St. Francis. She is only one of a great company of saints that have modeled the holiness of compassionate service. There is even an Archangel, Raphael, who is considered a bringer of healing.

Please share any thoughts or wisdom from your experience as a Spiritual Guide and a Benedictine Oblate. What resources do you recommend?

Caregivers can greatly benefit from regularly meeting with a group or a spiritual companion (spiritual director) for spiritual and emotional support. It can be such a help to periodically have a safe person or group to be with that will listen to you non-judgmentally and help you sort out the various demands, feelings, and hopes that are present in your life—and in the midst of that sorting-through of experiences listening for the subtle sacred invitation to discover a path of greater health and wholeness.

A spiritual guide (whether in an individual or group setting) should be able to help you explore your deepest truths and assist you in identifying practices that honor your spiritual life.

As a spiritual director, I normally meet with a directee once a month for an hour. We continue to meet as long as the directee wishes—often for years. We meet as two people sitting together listening for God's love and path of grace in the particular circumstances of the directee's life.

I am also an oblate with a Benedictine monastery in Three Rivers, Michigan. An "oblate" has taken vows to be supportive of the particular monastic community and to represent the spirituality of St. Benedict and the Benedictine Rule in the world. St. Benedict was one of the great founders of Western monasticism in the sixth century of the common era and established a monastic "Rule" or way of framing a Christian community based on gospel living.

Chapter 36 of the Rule of St. Benedict is devoted to concern for the community's care of its sick brothers or sisters. Benedict's guidance is both deeply grounded in holy scripture and in practical practices that keep relationships healthy and whole. This chapter reads in part:

Care of the sick must rank above and before all else so that they may truly be served as Christ, who said: "I was sick and you visited me" (Matthew 25:36) and, "What you did for the least of my people you did for me"

(Matthew 25:40). Let the sick on their part bear in mind that they are served out of honor for God, and let them not by their excessive demands distress anyone who serves them. Still, the sick must be patiently borne with, because serving them leads to a greater reward. Consequently, the prioress or abbot should be extremely careful that they suffer no neglect. (RB 36)

In Benedict's view, caring for someone who is sick is an opportunity to minister to Jesus Christ! There is no separating of the spiritual from the physical needs here. Caregiving is a spiritual practice as much as it is a physical practice.

And yet, there is a request for the sick person to take care not to be excessive in his or her demands. Benedictine spirituality has that quality of being both spiritual and practical, recognizing the sacred in the ordinary—and that is what I find compelling as a spirituality for our time.

http://llministries.homestead.com

Appendix 3

We Welcome You to Munchkin Land:
Inspirational Stories from Other Survivors

My Experience with ALS

By S. W. Hawking

I am quite often asked: How do you feel about having ALS? The answer is, not a lot. I try to lead as normal a life as possible, and not think about my condition, or regret the things it prevents me from doing, which are not that many.

It was a great shock to me to discover that I had motor neurone disease. I had never been very well co-ordinated physically as a child. I was not good at ball games, and my handwriting was the despair of my teachers. Maybe for this reason, I didn't care much for sport or physical activities. But things seemed to change when I went to Oxford, at the age of 17. I took up coxing and rowing. I was not Boat Race standard, but I got by at the level of inter-College competition.

In my third year at Oxford, however, I noticed that I seemed to be getting more clumsy, and I fell over once or twice for no apparent reason. But it was not until I was at Cambridge, in the following year, that my father noticed, and took me to the family doctor. He referred me to a specialist, and shortly after my 21st birthday, I went into hospital for tests.

I was in for two weeks, during which I had a wide variety of tests. They took a muscle sample from my arm, stuck electrodes into me, and injected some radio opaque fluid into my spine, and watched it going up and down with x-rays, as they tilted the bed. After all that, they didn't tell me what I had, except that it was not multiple sclerosis, and that I was an a-typical case.

I gathered however, that they expected it to continue to get worse, and that there was nothing they could do, except give me vitamins. I could see that they didn't expect them to have much effect. I didn't feel like asking for more details, because they were obviously bad.

The realisation that I had an incurable disease, that was likely to kill me in a few years, was a bit of a shock. How could something like that happen to me? Why should I be cut off like this?

However, while I had been in hospital, I had seen a boy I vaguely knew die of leukaemia, in the bed opposite me. It had not been a pretty sight. Clearly, there were people who were worse off than me. At least my condition didn't make me feel sick. Whenever I feel inclined to be sorry for myself, I remember that boy.

Not knowing what was going to happen to me, or how rapidly the disease would progress, I was at a loose end. The doctors told me to go back to Cambridge and carry on with the research I had just started in general relativity and cosmology. But I was not making much progress, because I didn't have much mathematical background. And, anyway, I might not live long enough to finish my PhD.

I felt somewhat of a tragic character. I took to listening to Wagner, but reports in magazine articles that I drank heavily are an exaggeration. The trouble is once one article said it, other articles copied it, because it made a good story. Anything that has appeared in print so many times, must be true.

My dreams at that time were rather disturbed. Before my condition had been diagnosed, I had been very bored with life. There had not seemed to be anything worth doing.

But shortly after I came out of hospital, I dreamt that I was going to be executed. I suddenly realized that there were a lot of worthwhile things I could do if I were reprieved. Another dream that I had several times, was that I would sacrifice my life to save others. After all, if I were going to die anyway, it might as well do some good.

But I didn't die. In fact, although there was a cloud hanging over my future, I found to my surprise, that I was enjoying life in the present more than before. I began to make progress with my research, and I got engaged to a girl called Jane Wilde, who I had met just about the time my condition was diagnosed.

That engagement changed my life. It gave me something to live for. But it also meant that I had to get a job if we were to get married. I therefore applied for a research fellowship at Gonville and Caius (pronounced Keys) College, Cambridge. To my great surprise, I got a fellowship, and we got married a few months later.

The fellowship at Caius took care of my immediate employment problem. I was lucky to have chosen to work in theoretical physics, because that was one of the few areas in which my condition would not be a serious handicap. And I was fortunate that my scientific reputation increased, at the same time that my disability got worse. This meant that people were prepared to offer me a sequence of positions in which I only had to do research, without having to lecture.

We were also fortunate in housing. When we were married, Jane was still an undergraduate at Westfield College in London, so she had to go up to London during the week. This meant that we had to find somewhere I could manage on my own, and which was central, because I could not walk far. I asked the College if they could help, but was told by the then Bursar: it is College policy not to help Fellows with housing. We therefore put our name down to rent one of a group of new flats that were being built in the market place. (Years later, I discovered that those flats were actually owned by the College, but they didn't tell me that.)

However, when we returned to Cambridge from a visit to America after the marriage, we found that the flats were not ready. As a great concession, the Bursar said we could have a room in a hostel for graduate students. He said, "We normally charge 12 shillings and 6 pence a night for this room. However, as there will be two of you in the room, we will charge 25 shillings." We stayed there only three nights.

Then we found a small house about 100 yards from my university department. It belonged to another College, who had let it to one of its fellows. However he had moved out to a house he had bought in the suburbs. He sub-let the house to us for the remaining three months left on his lease. During those three months, we found that another house in the same road was standing empty.

A neighbour summoned the owner from Dorset, and told her that it was a scandal that her house should be empty, when young people were looking for accommodation. So she let the house to us. After we had lived there for a few years, we wanted to buy the house, and do it up. So we asked my College for a mortgage. However, the College did a survey, and decided it was not a good risk. In the end, we got a mortgage from a building society, and my parents gave us the money to do it up.

We lived there for another four years, but it became too difficult for me to manage the stairs. By this time, the College appreciated me rather more, and there was a different Bursar. They therefore offered us a ground floor flat in a house that they owned. This suited me very well, because it had large rooms and wide doors. It was sufficiently central that I could get to my University department, or the College, in my electric wheel chair. It was also nice for our three children, because it was surrounded by garden, which was looked after by the College gardeners.

Up to 1974, I was able to feed myself, and get in and out of bed. Jane managed to help me, and bring up the children, without outside help. However, things were getting more difficult, so we took to having one of my research students living with us. In return for free accommodation, and a lot of my attention, they helped me get up and go to bed.

In 1980, we changed to a system of community and private nurses, who came in for an hour or two in the morning and evening. This lasted until I caught pneumonia in 1985. I had to have a tracheostomy operation. After this, I had to have 24-hour nursing care. This was made possible by grants from several foundations.

Before the operation, my speech had been getting more slurred, so that only a few people who knew me well, could understand me. But at least I could communicate. I wrote scientific papers by dictating to a secretary, and I gave seminars through an interpreter, who repeated my words more clearly.

However, the tracheostomy operation removed my ability to speak altogether. For a time, the only way I could communicate was to spell out words letter by letter, by raising my eyebrows when someone pointed to the right letter on a spelling card. It is pretty difficult to carry on a conversation like that, let alone write a scientific paper.

However, a computer expert in California, called Walt Woltosz, heard of my plight. He sent me a computer program he had written, called Equalizer. This allowed me to select words from a series of menus on the screen, by pressing a switch in my hand. The program could also be controlled by a switch, operated by head or eye movement. When I have built up what I want to say, I can send it to a speech synthesizer.

At first, I just ran the Equalizer program on a desk top computer. However, David Mason, of Cambridge Adaptive Communication, fitted a small portable computer and a speech synthesizer to my wheel chair. This system allowed me to communicate much better than I could before. I can manage up to 15 words a minute. I can either speak what I have written, or save it on disk. I can then print it out, or call it back, and speak it sentence by sentence.

Using this system, I have written a book, and dozens of scientific papers. I have also given many scientific and popular talks. They have all been well received. I think that is in a large part due to the quality of the speech synthesizer, which is made by Speech Plus.

One's voice is very important. If you have a slurred voice, people are likely to treat you as mentally deficient: Does he take sugar? This synthesizer is by far the best I have heard, because it varies the intonation, and doesn't speak like a Dalek. The only trouble is that it gives me an American accent. However, the company is working on a British version.

I have had motor neurone disease for practically all my adult life. Yet it has not prevented me from having a very attractive family, and being successful in my work. This is thanks to the help I have received from Jane, my children, and a large number of other people and organisations. I have been lucky that my condition has progressed more slowly than is often the case. But it shows that one need not lose hope.

Interview with Robin Cohn,
A TBI Survivor and Vice President of the New York State
Brain Injury Association

When did you suffer TBI? Please describe the accident(s) and how long it took you to realize you were injured.

I suffered my TBI in a car accident on June 19, 1996. I was rear-ended while stopped, and waiting to make a left turn. I was smashed into the car in front of me.

The seatbelt tightened around my neck, and it was very hard for me to breathe. I was able to slide my hand down to release the belt, and fell over onto the armrest. I felt like I was detached from my body. My head felt like it was filling with water, my eyes could not focus and the right side of my body felt tingly and numb. I knew I was badly injured when I could not sit back up.

I then drifted off into what felt like a very deep sleep. It was very hard to stay awake, many people were surrounding me and they seemed to be moving in slow motion. I could not understand their questions; it was so hard to think! My tongue felt very heavy, my mouth was difficult to move, and it was so hard to speak. I really needed to sleep.

What kind of symptoms did you notice from your TBI? How did these symptoms affect your life and self-esteem?

For weeks following the crash, even though I was told that the MRI was negative, and that I had suffered a very severe concussion, and that "all would eventually be well," I was still not feeling like myself.

It was as though my brain was made out of rubber. I could not absorb or process simple information. I was painfully fatigued all of the time. I could not concentrate, think clearly, and find the words I wanted to say. I said the wrong words for familiar items, could not sequence, alternate attention, multi-task, or remember anything.

I would get in the shower and forget what I was supposed to be doing in there! I would forget the steps to showering, and would get out with shampoo still in my hair. I felt like I was sleepwalking. I would sit in front of the mirror, wondering where I had gone. I looked like the same person, but I did not feel like myself.

This disconnected self of mine was having a difficult time trying to explain to those around me, why I just wasn't "snapping out of it," like they wanted me to. This was affecting every aspect of my life, and I was feeling so desperate for someone to help me!

How did TBI affect your job?

I attempted to go back to my work as a Dental Hygienist, which I had done for twenty-five years. I could not find my way to the office I had worked at for six years! I could not figure out how to do my job, set up my instruments, or what to even do with my instruments. I could not stay on schedule, had patients backing up in the waiting room, and was dropping instruments a lot, as I had tremendous weakness and numbness on the entire right side of my body. My capable hands were now of no use to me in my profession. I was desperate to make it look like I was capable, but the severe fatigue and mental confusion overpowered me.

I was quickly losing my self-esteem and confidence. My friends and family could not comprehend what on earth was wrong with me, and they soon began to lose their patience with me.

My boss suggested to me that I go home and take care of myself, because he was worried about me unintentionally causing harm to my patients. He replaced me with a temporary hygienist, and after a few months of me still not getting better, he permanently replaced me. I was devastated. Not only had my life turned upside down, but now I had lost the profession and the job I had loved so much.

What kinds of traditional treatment options did you try, and what, if any, help did these treatments provide?

It was recommended that I go for Chiropractic Treatment, Physical Therapy, Occupational Therapy, as well as taking a wide assortment of various pain and anti-depressant medications. The therapies were of a temporary help, and the meds seemed to either cause me more confusion, or fatigue, making the symptoms they were supposed to help, much worse! It was finally time for me to seek alternative therapies.

When and how did you discover yoga?

Luckily, my physician is very open-minded and into alternative therapies and treatments. She had been encouraging me to get involved in some gentle movement, and urged me to try yoga. I finally did so in 2000, and have been hooked on it ever since! It has been an amazing help in my recovery!

Are/were there any specific **asanas** *(positions) that provided relief from your symptoms or pain? Please describe how yoga helped your physical recovery from TBI.*

I began with a beginner's gentle yoga class, where I slowly started to get atrophied muscles moving once again. The more I went, the better I began to feel.

Over time, I challenged myself to a Level 1 class, and slowly began to notice a sense of increased mobility. Just simple cat and dog postures were almost too painful to bear at first, but working at a slow pace and staying determined, allowed me eventually to feel more stable in *asanas* that had initially been a great challenge for me.

The use of controlled breathing combined with simple asanas, brought me such an increased sense of wellbeing and better flexibility, in time.

Emotionally, mentally and spiritually, what differences did you notice? Please describe if/how yoga helped place your TBI into a broader context.

Over time, as my body started responding to the movement and increased flexibility the yoga brought me, I began to feel like I was moving forward in my healing. I found that my sense of self-esteem and confidence increasing as I combined movement and breath. I was opening my heart, body and spirit, to a new delight that was allowing space within my soul, for healing to take place—as I realized that I really needed to heal from the inside out.

Not only had my brain and external body been terribly injured, but so had my soul. The essence of who I truly was, once again started to emerge. Over time, through my spiritual awakening, I have come to view my "accident" as no accident at all. It has in fact allowed me the opportunity to be in touch with a part of myself that I had always been too busy and too preoccupied to delve into and nurture.

What motivated your decision to help teach yoga? How are you using your experience with TBI and yoga to help others recover from TBI?

My love of yoga of the last several years made me very interested in becoming a yoga instructor, so I could share my journey with others. I did attempt yoga teacher training recently (2005), but my cognitive deficits and fatigue made the hope of completing the training too challenging for me.

Instead, I assist a yoga teacher in a class that I started for TBI survivors from a day treatment facility. I may not be able to be a certified instructor, but it does not mean I cannot work with a teacher to allow others to experience the joys of yoga! These students are so thrilled to have the opportunity to be practicing yoga and reaping the wonderful benefits of asana and pranayam (breathing).

How/when did you become a Board Member of the New York State Brain Injury Association? Has this helped your TBI activism?

During my long and exhausting search for someone to help me find my way out of my TBI nightmare, I eventually got connected to the NYS Brain Injury Association. I received a lot of good information and assistance, and decided to get as involved as I could. I had an intense need to tell my story and to be heard. I wanted so much to be an advocate for others who were equally lost and uncertain of their futures as I was.

I immersed myself in their programs, conferences and committees, volunteering and attending as many events as I could. In time, I got involved in their Mentor Partnership Program, where I became a mentor to people who were new to brain injury.

I love being able to offer assistance and guidance to TBI patients and their loved ones. I do so with an open heart and lots of compassion for their situations. I always wish that I had had a mentor to help me through my long and difficult journey.

I also became involved in the BIANYS Speaker's Group, where I would talk to health care professionals about the effects of TBI. I became a Board Member of BIANYS two years ago. This is a bit challenging for me as I can get very overloaded at the meetings.

However, I do have a lot to offer with being a TBI survivor. I will continue to always be an advocate and am so happy that I had the courage to become so involved.

Have you seen other TBI survivors transform their lives through yoga as well?

As I mentioned previously, I began a yoga class for TBI survivors from the BIANYS day treatment center. The happiness, tranquility and peace that yoga brings to them is so rewarding! Their smiles just say so much about how happy they are to be practicing.

I am also on the Board of Directors for the Albany Kripalu Yoga Center, and as a chairperson of their outreach program, we have not only begun this class, but we have granted scholarships for TBI survivors who are interested in taking a session of various yoga classes. This allows those who perhaps would not be able to afford classes to do so!

What specific advice would you give to someone with TBI who is considering yoga?

My advice would be to not be afraid to try it. There is a class for every ability and every body. They need to know that yoga is done at one's own pace. There is no competition or judging, and the benefits of practicing yoga are amazing! The connection of body, mind and spirit is such a beautiful gift . . . one that everybody should experience!

Living and Hopeful with TBI

By Terri Nelson, Broadcast Editor

A guy with Alzheimer's who wasn't supposed to be driving got the keys and went for a ride on the night of November 20, 2004. He ran a red light and the cops said he was going 45 or 50 mph when he broadsided my car in the driver's door.

I was walking and talking after the crash but felt very odd. The rescue squad put me on a backboard and off we went in an ambulance. Once the X-rays established that my neck wasn't broken and I answered correctly what year it was and who was president of the U.S., the ER doc sent me home.

A day and a half later, a friend found me on my kitchen floor gushing blood out of my nose and mouth and I was headed back to the ER in an ambulance. They did a CT scan that time, but didn't find any "major damage."

Over the next couple of days, I lost my ability to read, couldn't stand light or noise, couldn't focus on anything and couldn't finish my sentences because the words just wouldn't come. I couldn't figure out how to do simple things like put on my pants or boil water for tea.

A friend recommended a doctor who had experience with concussions and she diagnosed me with post concussive syndrome. Based on my symptoms and how I described what I remembered about how my head banged around in the crash, she determined that I suffered diffuse axonal injury, with the most damage in the left-brain.

I ran out of sick time and went back to my job in three weeks as an editor for a newsgathering organization. I have a brain injury and I am a broadcast editor. How strange is that? I have gradually improved, but have struggled somewhat in my job.

My recovery has happened in spurts and plateaus. It seems miraculous sometimes and maddeningly inconsistent, too.

- I can get through a day at my very demanding job, but a trip down the cereal aisle in the grocery store can put me into a fog.
- I can play drums, but I put dog food in the coffeemaker.
- I can drive but when I'm on overload, I couldn't begin to tell anyone how to get from my home to my office and back again.
- I can feel good one day, but if I get too much visual stimulation, it can bring head pain and fogginess.

My recovery took a quantum leap forward in the summer of 2007 when I became part of a study in Charlottesville, Virginia. Sandy Rakowitz and

Robin Bernhard wanted to see how TTouch would benefit people with brain injuries and other neurological conditions. The study included sessions learning TTouch techniques and we have had EEGS to map the results.

After several months of this non-invasive work, I found that my head pain had decreased significantly, especially areas of visual stimulation and multi-tasking. The fog dissipated somewhat and my thought processes felt sharper. I found myself speaking better, with less difficulty in word-finding. TTouch is painless, simple and easy to do. It is also very calming.

Among the things I've learned about living with a brain injury is that I've had to learn my limits and adjust my life to fit them, not the other way around. For example, I don't go grocery shopping at the end of a workday and if I want to go to a movie theater or a concert, I realize that it might take a couple of days to recover from the visual and auditory stimulation. Or I can wear sunglasses and earplugs to the theater.

One of the most important things I've learned is to connect with others who've suffered brain injuries. Doctors really can't tell us much about our injuries, because every brain injury is different and because they can't explain what they haven't experienced.

I found that connecting with someone online, in a support group, or through word-of-mouth helped me find people who were having some of the same issues as me. Before I talked to others with similar symptoms, I felt unique, alone and somewhat crazy. There are a lot of us who share the same frustrations at the challenges and the same elation at our improvements.

Rising of the Phoenix

By Sandra K. Heggen—Fibromyalgia Survivor

In my 50th year, I died. Oh, there was no traveling through a tunnel, no bright white light, no floating above my body, none of the fun stuff. At least, I don't remember any of this sort of thing. But I don't remember dying, either. So, you wonder, how do I know I died? Well, I sort of figured it out later. Then you ask, how did you get to this death scene?

We'll have to go back a ways, nearly 15 years before my death. I'd always taken my physical health and strength for granted. Then I got this idea into my head that I needed to shape up. I started a program of running, eventually competing in marathons as well as lots of shorter races. I consulted with experts on diet and complementary types of exercises like strength training. I did all the things we're told we should do: I was de-fatted, de-salted, de-sugared, and de-caffeinated. I even meditated and did Tai Chi. I did all this along with my full time job as well as attending part-time university classes and participating in a navy reserve medical unit. For a time all seemed just fine. I was young and strong so why shouldn't I be able to do it all?

After a while, I noticed that the usual aches after running no longer went away, even after a good night's sleep. Then I realized that I rarely had a good night's sleep any more. I would wake in the middle of the night and be unable to get back to sleep. My weight started creeping up in spite of my diet and intense exercise. Achy stiffness inexorably spread from my legs and lower back to the rest of my body. Now it was with me all day, every day, slowly intensifying over the years. I developed an increasing fatigue that lingered even after weeks of vacations. But I was strong and healthy, right? Because I was doing all the right things. All I had to do was cut back a bit on my activity and give my body a chance to recover, right? Well, I guess I was wrong.

In addition, I experienced many stresses during this time. There was major surgery, several personal losses by deaths, increasing job pressures, then a job promotion and helping to prepare my reserve unit for deployment during Desert Storm. Finally, after years of increasingly futile struggle, it all culminated in a major crash-and-burn, a total physical, mental and emotional collapse. I had to take early retirement on disability. Exhausted, I simply sat in my recliner all day, in constant pain all over, unable to think a clear thought, emotionally distraught because I didn't know what was happening to me and why. How could I have been so betrayed? And by whom? I'd done all the right things, hadn't I?

That's when I died. I think. One clear memory I have is of sitting in my recliner, head back, eyes closed and actually groaning aloud, even though nobody else was in the house, "I can't do this any more!" As near as I can tell, nothing happened, but I could be wrong. Again.

My intellectual stance took a sharp turn from the analytical, left-brained activities I'd been so good at for so long. Over the next 10 years I made changes in my diet, paying attention to what my body wanted even if that didn't agree with "all the right things." I experimented with alternative therapies, some of which gave a bit of relief and some that apparently did nothing. My weight gain continued while my ability to walk without pain worsened. Nevertheless, at this point my overall body pains are less and I feel better emotionally and psychically. If someone would ask me, I'd say I'm healthy. Go figure.

But, you ask impatiently, how do you know you died? I'm getting to that. You know how, when you call up the memory of an event or a dream, you not only recall it, you remember doing the deed or having the dream? Well, did you ever have a memory of something you never did and that you never dreamt? No? I did. A few years ago, without warning, this "memory" popped into my head. I'm coming up on a group of five or six people wearing long robes and I'm saying, "I'm home! I'm home!" I'm so overcome with emotion I can hardly breathe or speak. The enveloping feelings of welcome and love are so achingly intense that I can't describe them. Believe me when I tell you, I've never felt anything like that in this world.

I was perplexed because I couldn't account for such a memory. It kept recurring—and being pushed away—at odd times, then one day, I got exasperated and decided to give it some attention. To my amazement, I discovered that those weren't people. Now this is where it gets really weird. They were balls of sparkling blue energy, sort of like Fourth of July sparklers, with diaphanous white vapor-like wisps trailing beneath them.

There was still that emotional tone of overwhelming love and acceptance, though. Loving energy balls? Wooo! Now it gets weirder. At some point, I suddenly realized that if those people looked like that then I must look like that, too! By now I suppose you're bound to decide that this was a hallucination. You just have to take my word for it that this was completely different from a hallucination. Neither was it a dream. It was realer than real.

It was some time before I concluded that these "people" were souls who had greeted me on my return Home. Dumbfounded, I was then left with the question, when could this have happened? After all, here I was in this all too solid and voluminous flesh, and definitely not dead. Ultimately, I recollected how I had felt those years ago on my recliner, unable to "do it anymore," feeling like I would "die of tired." I would breathe out and have to remind myself to breathe in again even though I felt no urgent need to do so. I felt so tired, so sleepy, all my energy leaking out. Maybe I did "fall asleep" and breathe out and not breathe in again. I'll never know for sure. One thing I ask you to consider though: when was the last time you paid attention to your breath (meditation aside) and then actually remembered it ten years later? *No, this was not a normal breathing.*

If this is indeed what happened and I did die and go Home, it's pretty apparent I didn't stay. Maybe I just went for a visit to charge up my batteries, so to speak. Lack of tunnels and white lights notwithstanding, I do believe something like a near-death experience happened. After that is more or less when I began my spiritual search in earnest, even though I didn't become aware of the memory itself for many more years.

Recently I was discussing the myth of the phoenix with some people. While it's interesting, and even seems associated with my astrological sign (Scorpio), I didn't feel any visceral connection but I couldn't quite forget the discussion. Later, I was having one of those conversations, you know, the kind where you think you're having a mental chat with someone else but you're really talking to yourself. Anyway, I was "talking" about my crash and burn and I was saying that it was so severe that "there was nothing left but ashes." Bam! Blink. Light bulb! Crash and burn. Dying. Ashes. Phoenix. Ahh, yes.

So, where am I now? Well, I'm not dead. I'm sitting in my recliner, still with a greater or lesser degree of chronic pain, unable to walk more than several feet, even with a cane, and literally nearly twice the woman I used to be. Yet, after 20 years of symptoms and 10 years after I crashed and ashed, I'm different, more hopeful, more alive, happier, than when I was "healthy."

I'm rising out of my ashes.

An Interview with Sarah Kramer,
CFS Survivor and
Co-Author and Author of Three Bestselling Cookbooks

Please describe the symptoms and experiences leading up to your diagnosis with CFS.

I had a large amount of stress prior to falling ill. I had just broken up with my longtime boyfriend, I was working overtime to make up for the loss income, plus I was just an incredibly unhappy person who didn't have a lot of coping skills.

I didn't know what was happening to me. I felt like I was getting the flu, my body ached, I was dizzy, exhausted, I felt like my brain was wrapped in cotton (brain fog), I had no appetite, I had panic attacks, my muscles hurt, I became allergic to foods I had never had problems with before, I had chemical sensitivities, I could smell EVERYTHING (car fumes, perfume, the smell of an orange) and it all made me feel sick. I couldn't have a normal conversation if there was too much noise, I couldn't read anymore.

Every day was different. Every single day something else hurt or another symptom popped up or mysteriously went away. But it was the fatigue that was debilitating and most frightening to me. Sometimes lifting my arm to itch a scratch on my face was too difficult. I felt dead inside.

How long did it take from when you first noticed symptoms until you found someone who knew how to treat them?

This was over 10 years ago when I first got sick . . . and CFS sadly called The Yuppie Flu and not taken that seriously, so I was quickly shoved by my doctor at the time into a hypochondriac box.

Unsatisfied with his treatment I started shopping for a new doctor who would take me seriously. It took me about a year and approx 8-9 different doctors before I found a someone who would actually take the time to figure out what was going on with me and after a bazillion different tests he diagnosed me with CFS.

Were you ever able to locate a particular CFS trigger, or did the illness apparently "come out of nowhere"?

Well hindsight is everything and much later, after my CFS diagnosis we were able to put together some of the puzzle pieces. It was a combination of all the lifestyle stress I was having as well as being severely overexposed to chemicals. I was a hairdresser, I also worked in a darkroom with toxic chemicals, a few years previous I had been on antibiotics for about a year, due to a misdiagnosis by my doctor. I was completely unaware that my body was spiraling out of control.

The straw that broke my camel's back came in the form of a spider bite, or rather the medication my doctor gave me to help with my spider bite. "Take one before bed and one in the morning and the itching and swelling will go away." Like a good patient, I popped my pill and went to bed. I woke up groggy and sluggish. As I got ready for work I went about my morning routine like a sleepy zombie. I popped the last of my medication and headed out to walk to work.

As I progressed up the street to work I started to feel funny. Only a 10 minute walk away, as I progressively started to feel funnier and funnier I had a million thoughts racing through my head. What was wrong with me? Why did I feel like I was walking in a tunnel? Why could I smell everything? Why was everything so loud?

As I bumped into a friend on the street the conversation I had with him was so difficult. I felt like I was walking through a pool of molasses and talking to him was becoming increasingly difficult.

I managed to get into building I worked at and ran into the bathroom to sit down and try and get myself together. I knew something was drastically wrong, but couldn't figure out what was going on. I finally opened the stall and grabbed a woman by the sinks and somehow managed to get the words "Get help!" out before I passed out on the floor.

A reaction to Benadryl.

From that day forward, I was never the same. I became sensitive to chemicals, smells, lights, cold, food. I found it increasingly difficult to get out of bed. I would sometimes crawl to the bathroom because it was easier then walking.

I was falling apart and I was too young, inexperienced and too sick to find the help I needed.

My doctor thought I was just tired and told me to take a vacation or move back in with my parents. I knew something was wrong with me, so I sought a second opinion. He sent me to an ear, nose and throat guy, who sent me to an ear specialist, who sent me to another doctor who sent me to a shrink. Finally, after eight or nine different doctors I found a doctor who said "There is obviously something wrong with you, so let's figure this out."

Many test. Many, many tests later, the diagnosis was myalgic encephalomyelitis aka Chronic Fatigue Syndrome or The Yuppie Flu. At that time, there wasn't much information available and the internet wasn't something I had even heard of, so I stumbled down to the local library and read everything I could on CFS.

I found the lack of information really disheartening and the fact that I had an illness that nobody knew anything about really depressing. After months of fighting with my fatigue, my confusion, my panic attacks and all the other symptoms that go with CFS . . . A friend of mine took me to his naturopath and my life changed.

What I learned in the doctor's office was that **I was responsible for my health**. That I could either passively let these things happen to me or I could arm myself with a little knowledge and learn about the things that work to heal my body.

How long have you had CFS?

I was ill for about a year before my diagnosis but all together it's been about 13+ years or so.

What kinds of treatments did you try and how, if at all, were they effective?

I was so desperate to get my body back that I would try anything that was suggested to me. The first thing I had to do was quit my job and go on welfare briefly. There was no way I could work anymore. So with the help of a wonderful social worker I got disability welfare and used that time to concentrate on getting well. My job was now to heal my body. I did cold water therapy, color bath therapy, massage, yoga, lots of exercise, no exercising, I ate liver, I juiced, I napped, I saw a therapist.

For me I found that yoga, massage were very effective for my body and therapy was effective for my brain. Early on, I spent a lot of time in bed or on the couch resting, and the yoga kept me limber and the massage helped work out the pain in my muscles. The therapy helped me to deal with what I was going through.

I would do 15-20 minutes of yoga every single day. Not serious, tie yourself into a pretzel yoga, but simple yoga from a book I found at the library. I usually had a tiny window of energy in the afternoon and that's when I would do my yoga. I would then rest and do my visualization exercise. I would think of myself as rechargeable battery as I lay on the bed, and I would try and envision myself filling up with energy.

I also found that having one or two goals a day to very effective. At my worst I could barely get dressed, read, carry on a decent conversation. So every night I would think of one thing I wanted to do the next day. Whether it be get dressed, go for a walk, write a letter. It gave me a purpose, a reason to be proud of myself. I spent so much time lying around depressed because I felt like a waste of space and a burden.

These small things that I could accomplish once or twice a day gave me a feeling of worth. "I got dressed!" YAY!! It was the little things like that, which kept me going.

Also, removing allergens from my diet as well as changing my diet was very effective. I was raised Vegetarian, but it wasn't until I went Vegan and started really constructing healthy well rounded meals that I noticed a big increase in my energy level.

You are the author of three best-selling vegan cookbooks. Did your experience with CFS contribute in any way to your interest in a vegan diet and your interest in writing a cookbook? If so, how?

Well as a Vegan, I had a hard time finding Vegan cookbooks where the food actually tasted . . . good. *laugh* So my co-author and I started compiling recipes and the rest is history. But if it wasn't for my CFS, I don't think I would have taken an interest in really exploring Vegan eating and ways to make a Vegan diet interesting and tasty.

In your photos and writing, you seem like a bundle of energy. How do you manage to write new cookbooks, promote your published books, and balance your personal life—especially after having CFS?

Looks can be deceiving. Photoshop does wonders for bags under the eyes. *laugh* While I am not always a bundle of energy, I am always a bundle of ideas. So, I always have a notepad at hand and I am constantly writing down ideas, thoughts or plans to execute. I have had to create a life with my husband where I don't work a regular job. I work when I feel up to it. That's where being self-employed comes in handy. I can set my own hours, nap or take the day off when needed.

Plus, there are things I do every day to promote energy in myself. I don't use an alarm clock. I let my body sleep until it's ready to wake up. When I get that funny tired CFS feeling from doing too much, I'll go lay down.

I have my friends over, rather then going out, because I find all the noise of clubs and the stress of going out aggravates me. I exercise every day. I drink tons of water. I eat a healthy vegan diet. I meditate.

If I can't do something because of my CFS, I just figure out another way to approach it. Most importantly, I try to keep things as simple as possible.

Promotion of the cookbooks is difficult, because the stress of traveling really takes its toll on me. So, my publishers and I plan out my trips carefully, making sure I have enough time to rest, take a nap, have a day to lie around and re-charge in between my engagements. On my last book tour, my friend

Jen did all the driving while I napped in the back of the car. That really helped me to be fresh for the book signings.

I do usually fall apart once I get home, and I spend 3-4 days recuperating from my trip. It's a back and forth balancing act that has just become second nature.

When I was first ill, I was running at about 10%. I now feel like I'm at about 75-80%. But it wasn't just like one day I started feeling better. It's been a long gradual journey, discovering what works and what doesn't work for me.

For me, stress is the biggest trigger and in the last 4 or 5 years, I have made a large step forward with my CFS. I believe that part of it has been cleaning out my system and the other part has been cleaning out my life. *laugh*

Learning to let go of the stuff that doesn't matter. Letting go of the people who get me worked up and stressed out. Learning how to live a stress free life. I used to think I had to be all things to all people, and now I just have to be me. Finding a good balance in everything I do has been key.

Also, living with animals has taught me so much about healthy lounging. *laugh* My cats were instrumental in teaching me that laying around conserving energy is a good thing and my dog Fergus gets me up and around the block, even on days when I don't want to move.

Whom do you most admire and why?

My dog. He keeps it simple and I admire and strive for that.

What would you most like to share with other survivors?

I would like to share my five simple rules for survival.

1. **Listen to your body.** Even if you're not listening, it's telling you something. If you're tired. Rest. If you're sad. Cry. Don't fight it. Be selfish. Or, as I like to say, "Self-Full." Take care of yourself first and everything else will fall into place.
2. **You know your body best**. Even when everyone else (doctors, friends, family etc) are telling you different. If there's a voice inside your head that's telling you different . . . go with that voice. You are the only one who knows how you feel.
3. **Knowledge is power**. Educate yourself on your illness.
4. **Doctors are like shoes**. You have to try on a few before you find the one that fits. Don't be afraid to ask questions, especially if you have a little knowledge that the doctor doesn't seem to have (see #3).

5. **Food is fuel.** Without a healthy diet, your body will fall apart, no matter who you are. If you can learn what helps to create a healthy body and arm yourself with the knowledge to make it strong, you will be powerful. There will be no stopping you.

What does "The Wizard of Oz" mean to you?

Well for starters, it was my favourite movie when I was a kid. It was a family event every year to watch it when it aired at Christmas time. We had a black and white TV and my Dad would show me how the black and white would become "better quality" when Dorothy left Kansas to go to Oz. It wasn't until high school that I realized the movie was in color. *laugh*

Today, it is still one of my all time favourite movies. Now as an adult who has lived through a major health crisis, the message of the movie is much more clear to me. At the end of the movie, Dorothy states:

"If I ever go looking for my heart's desire again, I won't look any further than my own backyard."

To me that means you have a choice to make. You can run around Oz asking everyone to help you. Or you can look inside yourself because the strength and energy you need is already there. You just have to have the "brains," "courage" and "heart" to look inside.

Sarah Kramer appears courtesy of *www.GoVegan.net*

What the Mythological Figure of Kali
Can Teach Us about Overcoming Trauma

By Laura Bruno,
TBI Survivor and Life Coach

Black and naked (except for a necklace of 50 human heads)—hair wild and tongue out, Kali certainly knows how to make an entrance! Brandishing a sword and a human head in her two left hands, she destroys everything in her path and then dances maniacally upon the dead. In terror, awe and morbid fascination, we stare. Fight or flight?

But how can we fight she who destroyed everything we thought we knew? Cut to the core, how can we run? No matter: in a battle against the universe itself, *where* would we run? Old instincts flare, but they no longer serve. When Kali appears, life as we knew it ceases to exist.

As a Medical Intuitive and Life Coach specializing in transitions, I receive many "post-Kali" calls. Individual traumas vary: life-threatening illness, disabling injury, divorce, job loss, natural disaster, financial emergency, or—sometimes even more disturbing—an uncanny sense that things are *about* to change. (Kali phones ahead with her party plans.)

Despite variations, these experiences hold one thing in common: they demand attention. What little warnings, gentle nudges, intuitive hits or lesser traumas did not accomplish, Kali has. Distractions, whether silly or sophisticated, just can't compete with complete annihilation.

In order to begin rebuilding, we first need to examine the destruction. Doing so takes courage. Even though we ultimately need to look at the mess ourselves, it helps to have a Kali-survivor involved in the surveying process. Someone who has already faced Kali knows the pain of loss in a way that well-meaning friends or family sometimes cannot understand.

There are losses and then there is what I call a "Kali loss": the sense that our entire reality was an illusion and nothing real remains. This feeling does not respond to typical cheer-up methods because those methods, too, reveal their illusory nature. Alone and scared, we yearn for deep, unchanging truth. Anything less just adds to the overwhelming carnage.

Most people cannot afford to witness this level of destruction because doing so might crumble their own comfortable sense of reality. Instinctively, they put up walls to protect themselves, fighting us when we try to share the magnitude of our experience. When our usual support system fails, we're supposed to turn inside, but inside's a terrifying mess right now.

We cry out to the universe for help and Kali herself arrives—in the form of someone who has already witnessed his or her own destruction and rebuilding. Someone who honors the beauty and life-giving force of such experiences. Someone who can afford to look at our mess because his or her reality has already crumbled and reassembled in a powerfully expansive way.

Non-attached to our previous conceptions or enculturations, s/he can more quickly and easily sift through the rubble, drawing our attention to pieces ready for new construction. S/he also helps us to look Kali in the face, recognizing our own prayers for change and ability to manifest the answers. When we paradoxically turn to Kali for help, she reveals herself not just as destroyer but as Mother-Creator.

Initially we might find Mother Kali in a book, a synchronous new friendship, a spiritual advisor, or Life Coach, but eventually we begin to recognize her in ourselves. By witnessing our own destruction, we find those parts that cannot be destroyed. We find our Essence, "that" which defies all labels and runs through everyone and everything.

Kali's black form absorbs all color and all vibration: she contains it all. The sword and head in her left hands symbolize Divine inspiration striking down our ego. The 50 human heads around her neck represent the 50 sounds of the Sanskrit alphabet—the root of all language. "In the beginning was the Word and the Word was with God and the Word was God." "But the Word is very near. It is in your mouth and in your heart so that you can do it." We feel Divinity surging through body, mind and spirit, and we, too, begin to dance. "Let the dead bury their own dead. Come, follow me."

Only then do we notice Kali's two right hands—ready to bestow the blessings. As a Mother, Kali does not shelter her children. She throws us into the fire and lets all illusion, enculturation and attachments burn to a crisp. We scream as costumes turn to ash, railing against a universe that allows such suffering.

And then it happens. We emerge from the fiery, bloodstained pit. Lighter, easier and full of Grace. We no longer fear death because we've already been through it. Signs of life sprinkle the horizon as green shoots push their way through now fertile soil. We learn that some trees will not plant seeds until the searing heat of fire tears through their casings.

Pain and sorrow reveal themselves as parts of *Life*. Freed from the limitations of fear and resistance, we can revel in naked existence. Recreating ourselves in ways that express the fullness of our being. When ego goes up in smoke, we turn ourselves inside out, and let our Light so shine. *Namaste.*

www.internationalrenaissancecoaching.com